Beyond Bikini Medicine

Diseases Affect Women Differently - How to Partner with Your Doctor for Better Outcomes.

Jyoti Patel, MD
EXPERT IN INTEGRATIVE & FUNCTIONAL MEDICINE

Copyright © 2025 by Dr. Jyoti Patel

All rights reserved.

No part of this book may be reproduced or transmitted in any form or by any means, electronic or mechanical, including photocopying, recording, or by any information storage and retrieval system, without permission in writing from the copyright holder, except for the use of brief quotations in a review.

This book is self-published by the author. For inquiries, contact:

www.JyotiPatelMD.com

Disclaimer:

This book is not intended as a substitute for professional medical advice. Consult your healthcare provider for personalized care.

ISBN: 979-8-3493-2726-1

Printed in the United States of America

First Edition May 2025

Dedication

To my sister, whose health scare ignited my mission to champion this cause. Your strength, resilience, and unwavering spirit continue to inspire me every day. This book is for you and for every woman who deserves to be heard and valued. Thank you for showing me that the fight for women's health is not just personal, it is a movement. I will dedicate my life to advocating for better care for all women, carrying forward the inspiration you have given me.

Contents

Author's Note 5

Disclaimer 7

Introduction - A Doctor's Journey Through the
Gender Gap in Medicine... 8

Part 1 - The Blueprint to a Woman's Body   13

    Chapter 1 - Understanding The Female Body   14

    Chapter 2 - Hormone Health   27

    Chapter 3 - Heart Health   49

    Chapter 4 - Brain Health   72

    Chapter 5 - Mental Health   96

    Chapter 6 - Immune Health   120

    Chapter 7 - Digestive Health   138

    Chapter 8 - Musculoskeletal Health   162

Part 2 - Beyond Knowledge: Turn Awareness into Action   188

    Chapter 9 - Speak Up: Communicating with Yourself and Your Doctor   189

    Chapter 10 - Own Your Health: Advocate, Share, and Empower Each Other   206

    Appendix A - The ACE Test   219

    Appendix B - Recommended Supplements for Lasting Health   224

    Appendix C - Women's Complete Health Resource Guide   240

About The Author 247

Endnotes 248

Author's Note

"I can't breathe, and I haven't slept all night. I can't lay down and I'm scared," my terrified sister cried over the phone. It was around the time of the pandemic, when I received this phone call that shook me to my core.

I instructed her to go immediately to the ER, assuring her I would meet her there. Racing into the ER, I was met by a doctor who had just finished running some tests. His demeanor was calm and dismissive, "All the tests are normal," he said. "I'm just waiting for the chest x-ray and then I will discharge her home".

I couldn't believe my ears.

What!?

Sending her home!?

I was livid. He seemed to dismiss her symptoms altogether, attributing them to stress, despite her growing discomfort.

As her sister and as a female medical doctor, I knew something was seriously wrong. I advocated fiercely for her, calling in specialists and pushing for further tests. Suddenly, I heard the loud beeping of the monitor behind me. As I turned towards my sister, I witnessed as she turned gray and collapsed back onto the gurney, slipping into cardiac arrest before my eyes. I watched in horror as the medical staff rushed in quickly to revive her. It was clear that they had missed something crucial. The doctor had been confident in his initial assessment—too confident. To me, it seemed as though he had dismissed her simply because she was young, female, and healthy. When he returned, he was surprised to learn that she had a cardiac issue, and he had missed it all along. After 200 ccs of fluid were removed from around her heart, a life-threatening condition known as tamponade, the surgeon was shocked, "She is young and healthy; this should not have happened".

One Size Does <u>Not</u> Fit All

For too long, medicine has relied on a one-size-fits-all approach, failing to recognize that this "size" was constructed around studies of men, leaving women to suffer the consequences. As a result, we shouldn't be surprised when our medical system fails to recognize heart symptoms in women when the textbook we use to diagnose and treat most diseases was not written for us in the first place!

As a female physician, it was not until this deeply personal experience with my sister that I truly understood the urgent need for change in women's healthcare. This experience opened my eyes to just how many women are dismissed or misdiagnosed because their symptoms do not fit the mold. If I had not been there to advocate for my sister, I wonder: Would she have received the care she needed?

I shudder to imagine how many other women have been ignored, their pain brushed aside, simply because the system has not caught up with the science on women's health. This disparity is not born from a lack of compassion; it stems from a lack of knowledge.

Break The Silence

This book is a call to action to advocate for yourself, to demand better care, and to reshape the medical system that has long failed women. It is time we break the silence surrounding women's health and challenge the way we view and treat diseases in women. I hope this book will empower you to take charge of your health and push for the care you deserve.

Disclaimer

The information in this book is intended to inform and empower you on your health journey. While it provides valuable insights, it is not meant to replace professional medical advice. Use the knowledge you gain here to begin an open and informed conversation with your healthcare provider. Always consult your doctor or healthcare team for any health concerns to ensure that your care is tailored to your specific needs. Your health is unique, and your provider is there to help guide you.

Introduction

A Doctor's Journey Through the Gender Gap in Medicine

Did you know, before 1993 women were excluded from most medical research?[1] For decades, the male body was considered the default in clinical trials. Medical treatments, diagnostic criteria, and even the "normal" ranges for lab tests were based entirely on men and then applied to women as if we were just smaller versions of them. Even though heart disease is the leading cause of death in women, 50% of women who are having a heart attack are sent home from the emergency room because their symptoms do not match the male-based standards we use in medicine.[2]

This reality hit close to home when my mother, the strong matriarch of our family known for her grit and resilience, began experiencing intermittent back pain. Despite seeking medical attention, her concerns were quickly dismissed as arthritis in her back. It was not until she collapsed while walking in the neighborhood that she was rushed to the hospital, where a 99% blockage in a heart artery was discovered, requiring an urgent cardiac stent. How many other women have lost their lives, or their lives have been changed forever because of this blind spot in medicine?

When I think about 1993, it was not that long ago. I was a young college student, encouraged by a science professor who saw something in me I had not yet seen in myself. "You should consider pre-med," he said, and his confidence lit a fire in me, launching my journey to becoming a physician. Like many young women of that time, I was focused on carving out my future, believing the world was open to us if we worked hard enough.

But here is what I did not know, while I was dreaming of helping people as a doctor, the medicine I was studying, the textbooks, the lectures, and the evidence-based protocols I would use to treat patients were largely built on research that excluded women. This was not just an oversight; it was a dangerous gap, one that created a massive misunderstanding of how diseases show up differently in women and how we respond to treatments. A grave misunderstanding that unknowingly cost countless lives.

During my Internal Medicine residency, we often deferred 'women's health concerns' to our OB/GYN colleagues, under the misconception that women's health was confined to breast and reproductive issues, a narrow view often referred to as 'Bikini Medicine.' This was not out of neglect, but rather a lack of awareness. We simply did not recognize that conditions like heart disease, digestive issues, autoimmune disorders, and even brain health issues could present differently in women. At the time, I did not question this approach, after all, this was what we were taught. I believed I was providing the best care possible, unaware of the gaps in my understanding.

But too often I witnessed, when women's symptoms didn't align with the male-centric models in our textbooks, they were dismissed as stress or anxiety. Doctors did not dig deeper, often because we lacked the tools and training to connect the dots between women's unique biology and the diseases they were experiencing. This blind spot has had profound consequences, leaving many women unheard, misdiagnosed, and underserved.

This discrepancy is glaringly obvious when it comes to heart disease as I realized with my own mother. Women often experience significant delays in diagnosis, with many sent home from the emergency room, misdiagnosed, or dismissed. Studies show that women are more likely to die from their first heart attack than men, a shocking reality we cannot ignore. Women also face worse outcomes from heart medications and procedures, because they were not tested in women.

Another example is that autoimmune diseases disproportionately affect women, with 80% of all cases occurring in females. However, it can take an average of six years for a woman to be diagnosed with lupus, a disease that increases the risk of heart disease five-fold and can cause serious damage to the kidneys, lungs, and brain.[3] Because our diagnostic criteria and treatment protocols are based on male physiology, there are delays in diagnosis, and this oversight leaves countless women at risk of preventable complications and long-term health damage.

And then there's Alzheimer's disease. Women make up two-thirds of all Alzheimer's patients, yet we still do not have enough female-focused brain studies to truly understand how to prevent or treat this devastating condition.[4]

Drug research has historically focused predominantly on men, ignoring the critical fact that women often respond differently to medications. The reality is that women's health has been sidelined in medical research, drug development, and safety testing. For years, medication dosages and efficacy were rarely studied in women, leaving a significant gap in our understanding of how these treatments truly affect half the population.[5]

I once asked my sister and brother-in-law, both pharmacists, if they were taught in pharmacy school that men and women respond differently to medications. Their answer? "No." I was floored. And here's another embarrassing truth, most medical schools do not teach it either. Can you believe that? Doctors are not routinely trained to consider that women might need different doses, medications, or treatments because our bodies process and store drugs in ways that are unique to us.

And it gets worse. Women are more likely to experience severe side effects or even harm from medications. In fact, 80% of the drugs pulled off the market due to dangerous side effects were found to pose greater risks to women.[6] So, while we continue to trust the system, it is clear that women's health is too often an afterthought, leaving us to pay the price.

Throughout my journey in clinical practice, I came to a humbling realization, I was part of a system built around male-centric standards. However, as I began to uncover the depth of these gender differences, I saw an opportunity to be part of the solution. To truly care for my female patients, I knew I had to move beyond the outdated frameworks that have long shaped medicine. This awareness became the driving force behind my work today, advocating for a more inclusive approach to women's health, one that acknowledges our unique needs extend far beyond Bikini Medicine.

While recognizing that gender is a complex and diverse concept, I will use "female" and "male" in this context to refer specifically to biological and chromosomal differences. This is to address the unique health needs based on sex while respecting the experiences of all individuals, including cisgender, bisexual, and transgender people.

Why This Book Matters

This book matters because there is hope. Hope that begins with awareness. It starts with recognizing that diseases affect men and women differently. It begins by empowering women to advocate for their own health, educating healthcare professionals on these critical gender differences, and demanding more gender-specific research, particularly for conditions that disproportionately affect women. My goal is to ignite a conversation and inspire a movement toward a transformative approach to women's health.

The good news is that we are making progress. Below are some key milestones in the evolution of this shift:
- **Pre-1990s**: Most clinical trials excluded women due to concerns about the impact of hormonal fluctuations and the belief that men's physiology was a more stable baseline.

- **1993**: The NIH Revitalization Act mandated that women and minorities be included in clinical research.
- **1994**: The FDA issued guidelines (though compliance was inconsistent) that tried to encourage the inclusion of women in clinical trials and the analysis of data by sex.
- **2000s**: Increased efforts were made to ensure sex differences were considered in clinical research, with the NIH emphasizing the importance of analyzing data by sex and gender.
- **2016**: The NIH introduced a policy requiring both male and female subjects to be included in preclinical research, with sex differences considered in study design and analysis.[7]

While significant strides have been made, the future of women's health is full of promise. As you read through the chapters that follow, remember that this is not just a book about women's health, it is a roadmap to a more personalized, effective, and empowering approach to your health. It is about recognizing that you are a unique individual with specific needs that deserve to be acknowledged and addressed.

Part 1

The Blueprint to a Woman's Body

Chapter 1
Understanding The Female Body

"Men Are from Mars, Women Are from Venus."

—**John Gray**

I remember when the life-changing book *Men Are from Mars, Women Are from Venus* came out in the '90's. I was a young college student learning to navigate new relationships, and this book made me realize why I struggled to understand the opposite sex. It was like a lightbulb moment— *That is why he did that?* It got me thinking about how men and women are different in how we feel, react, and deal with emotions. Now, years later, the truth is obvious: men and women are different! So why, in medicine, do we expect a one-size-fits-all approach to treating diseases in men and women?

Here we are, thirty years later, and medicine still treats men and women like they are the same. The male body has been the blueprint for human health for far too long. Before the '90's, women were left out of most medical research, clinical trials, and even medical textbooks, which were all focused on male physiology. Focusing only on how diseases affect men completely misses the mark because it ignores the deep and important differences in how diseases affect women, differences that go far beyond our reproductive organs.

As a doctor, I have learned that the same symptoms do not always mean the same thing, the same treatments do not work the same way, and the same health standards do not apply to everyone. Women are not just smaller versions of men. Our bodies work differently, whether it is how we process medications, how diseases show up, or how treatments affect us. This blind spot in medicine is not just frustrating, it is dangerous. It has cost lives and permanently changed others.

To drive this point home, let us flip the script.

Now, imagine landing on the planet Venus, where everything is flipped. The entire medical system is built around the female body. We only study heart disease in women and use the same diagnostic criteria, medications, and dosages on men. However, since men do not experience heart disease the same way or have the same risk factors, they are either misdiagnosed or treated too late. The result? Fifty percent of men die from their first heart attack. Can you even imagine the outrage? Men would be demanding immediate changes to the medical system.

So, why aren't we outraged when this is exactly what happens to women? Fifty percent—*half*—of the women having a heart attack are turned away from emergency rooms because their symptoms do not match the "male model" of heart disease.[8][9] Women are also more likely to die from their first heart attack compared to men.[10] The problem is: we do not know what we do not know. Most of us have no idea, even those of us practicing medicine (and yes, that includes female physicians), that the medical system we trust is beautifully designed for a man and poorly fitted for a woman.

Before we go further, I want to acknowledge an important consideration.

As I write this book, I want to acknowledge that gender holds diverse and deeply personal meanings within our culture, and I approach this diversity with both respect and compassion. In this work, however, I will focus on the biological distinctions between males and females as defined by genetic makeup and sex chromosomes, specifically XX and XY. While rare, some women may have a mix of cells with different chromosomal compositions due to conditions such as Turner syndrome (45X) or mosaicism (e.g., 46XX and 46XY). Additionally, racial differences in health risks and outcomes for women exist. By centering the discussion on the XX female as a whole, we can examine how these biological differences shape the health of the majority of females through a scientific perspective.

Men and women are different down to each one of our 37 trillion cells.[11]

Imagine putting on special goggles and zooming into your body. You would see organs made of tissues, tissues made of cells, and inside each cell, a nucleus containing chromosomes, your genetic blueprint. As women, every cell in our bodies has two X chromosomes, while men have one X and one Y. That second X chromosome does more than just play a role in reproduction; it shapes many aspects of who we are, from our brains to our bones.

If we are so different at the genetic level, down to every cell, why would we expect men and women to respond the same way to diseases or treatments? It does not make sense. Let us explore how our X chromosomes influence our health. It is a fascinating story written into our DNA, and it is one we need to understand.

Understanding our unique genetic makeup is just one piece of the puzzle. Our health is also deeply shaped by the natural rhythms that govern a woman's life, from month to month and season to season.

Women's Life Cycles Shape Health

Rhythm is life.

"We only have to dance to the rhythm of life."

—**Lailah Gifty Akita.**

During my third year of residency, my life had no rhythm. I was working long hospital shifts, surviving on Oreos and Diet Coke, and constantly sleep-deprived. Stress was my norm, and I was determined to power through no matter what. Then, the perfect storm hit. After I delivered my first child, I was diagnosed with cancer. At the time, I saw it as an inconvenience, not a crisis. My priority was finishing my training, so I ignored my body's need for rest and pushed forward. I underwent cancer surgery and radiation, assuming that was all that was needed for me to continue to strive and drive in my career. But I had a rude awakening when my PET scan the following year showed metastatic recurrence—cancer that had spread. This led to a second surgery, followed by another recurrence, requiring a third and then a fourth surgery.

It took me years to recognize the toll of my chaotic lifestyle, my lack of rhythm, and its impact on my health. I had been so focused on pushing through that I didn't realize how much my body needed balance, rest, nourishment, and care. That experience taught me a hard but invaluable lesson: rhythm is not optional. It is essential. Our bodies thrive on balance, and ignoring that truth comes at a cost. Now, I see that time as a turning point, one that reshaped how I approach health for myself and others.

For far too long, when we talk about rhythms and women's health, the focus has been narrowly placed on reproductive rhythms—what's often referred to as "bikini medicine." But you should know that our rhythms play a much bigger role in our overall health. Men do not have the same cyclical patterns due to their XY chromosomes, making their health experiences fundamentally unchanging and consistent. Our double X chromosomes, however, are the reason why we have daily, monthly, seasonal, and lifespan rhythms.

These natural cycles which include monthly hormonal changes, seasonal shifts, and life transitions like puberty, pregnancy, and menopause, profoundly impact heart health, brain function, cancer risk, and overall well-being. These rhythms are not just a part of life; they actively shape our health in ways that are unique to women. From the rollercoaster of puberty to the transformative shifts of menopause, these phases touch everything from our metabolism and brain function to our cardiovascular and bone health.

Every stage of life is influenced by these rhythms, and looking back, I can clearly see how deeply they have shaped me. I will never forget my teenage years, the hormonal pendulum swinging erratically leading to embarrassing acne, mood swings, food cravings, fatigue, and physical changes. It was a lot to navigate, and I often felt like I was just trying to keep up.

Then came adulthood, with its own set of rhythms. My cycles were more predictable, and I was better able to navigate the waves. I had this relentless drive and stamina that helped me juggle the chaos of work, relationships, and home life. I felt capable, even invincible at times, though I didn't always pause to appreciate it.

Now, in my 50s, I am in a whole new chapter. My metabolism has shifted, my sleep is not what it used to be, and even my mood feels different. The way I look, and the way I feel, it is all changing again, guided by the unique blueprint of my genetic code. And from talking to thousands of women over the years in the clinic, I know I am not alone in this. So many of us are navigating these changes, often without the guidance or understanding we deserve.

For women, fatigue, anxiety, digestive issues, pain, disconnection, and burnout are often rooted in being out of rhythm. We fall off the path of health when we push, strive, and drive ourselves, applauding productivity and intensity, while ignoring our cycles and seasons. Healing from chronic disease includes paying attention to the flow of life, rhythms, and circadian cycles.

Take our monthly menstrual cycle, or infradian cycle, unique in women that spans approximately 28 days and affects far more than just reproduction. This monthly rhythm impacts energy, mood, metabolism, and even how we respond to stress. In the first half of the menstrual cycle, rising estrogen boosts energy, focus, and recovery, making it a great time for high-intensity workouts, intermittent fasting and productivity. But as the cycle shifts, so do our needs, favoring rest, nourishing, nutrient-dense foods, and gentler activities during the luteal and menstrual phases. Learning to align our lifestyle with these rhythms in our younger years can be a game changer for both health and productivity.

And it is not just about menstrual cycles. Later life stages like pregnancy and menopause bring profound hormonal shifts that ripple through every system in the body. For instance, health issues during pregnancy, like high blood pressure, gestational diabetes, or pre-eclampsia, are unique risk factors for heart disease as we get older. And during menopause, the decline in estrogen does not just mark the end of reproduction; it affects our heart, bones, brain, metabolism, and even our gut microbiome, the trillions of bacteria, viruses, and fungi living in your gut.

With this foundation, you are ready to dive deeper.

In the chapters ahead, we are going to dive into seven key areas of women's health that I believe are essential for you to understand. Because knowledge is power when it comes to advocating for your health in the doctor's office. Each chapter will explore these topics in-depth, giving you the tools to take charge of your well-being. Here's a sneak peek to spark your curiosity and get you excited for what's to come.

CHAPTER 2 OVERVIEW

Hormones Are More Than Reproduction

"You are just hormonal' is a phrase often used in medicine to dismiss physical symptoms in women. While both men and women produce the same hormones, any unexplained symptoms in a woman are usually given a diagnosis of hormone issues. There are over fifty hormones in the female body, this kind of oversimplification does a major disservice to female health.[12] The truth is, hormones are complex and touch every organ system in the body, and understanding how they impact health can help us understand the real causes of diseases in women.

Women are especially attuned to hormonal rhythms that shift daily, monthly, seasonally, and across life stages. These fluctuations, influenced by stress, sleep, diet, movement, and emotions, impact blood pressure, blood sugar, metabolism, and even cancer risk.

To truly understand how hormones shape our health, we must move beyond reproductive labels and explore the broader hormonal ecosystem at work within us.

These hormones include, but are not limited to, estrogen, progesterone, testosterone, cortisol, insulin, thyroid hormones, and those that regulate appetite and metabolism. They are chemical messengers that our brain controls through specialized glands, sending signals to every cell in our body. They influence the function, flow, and rhythm of every cell, creating a complex web of communication that affects everything: energy, weight, sleep, mood, blood flow, blood sugar, memory, hunger, body temperature, and the health of our gut, bones, brain, and heart. This interconnectedness reminds us just how intricate and intelligent our physiology truly is.

In Chapter 2, we will dive deeper into how to regulate our hormones and explore the root causes behind the imbalances affecting them.

CHAPTER 3 OVERVIEW

Women's Heart Health, Not Just a Man's Game

Heart disease is perhaps one of the most critical topics I address in this book, as it remains the leading cause of death among women, accounting for one in every five female deaths. Yet many of us still think of it as a "man's disease." The truth is heart disease affects women differently. Our risk factors, symptoms, and even how we respond to treatments are unique. For example, women are more likely to experience subtle warning signs like fatigue, jaw pain, or nausea rather than classic chest pain. These differences mean we often go undiagnosed or misdiagnosed, sometimes until it is too late.

That is why understanding how heart disease shows up in women is lifesaving.

By understanding these nuances, recognizing early warning signs, and advocating for proactive screening, you can take charge of your heart health. In Chapter 3, we will explore how heart disease uniquely impacts women and discuss practical steps you can take to protect your heart and the hearts of the women you love. From nutrition and stress management to knowing your numbers, like blood pressure, cholesterol, and more, we will cover it all. Your heart is your lifeline, and it is time to give it the attention it deserves.

CHAPTER 4 OVERVIEW

Why Women's Brains Are at Risk

Did you know that women are at a significantly higher risk of developing Alzheimer's and dementia than men? Nearly two-thirds of those living with Alzheimer's are women.[13] This staggering statistic is not just a number; it is a call to action. Yet, dementia in women is often addressed too late, after the disease has already progressed, because symptoms are frequently dismissed. Women are told they are "just stressed" or casually joked with about "getting older," leaving many undiagnosed until significant damage has already occurred.

But what you may not know is that brain changes that lead to dementia often begin decades before symptoms appear, giving us the opportunity to intervene early and protect our cognitive health.

This is why this chapter is so vital. Understanding the unique risks women face when it comes to Alzheimer's and dementia can empower you to take proactive steps now to safeguard your brain health for the years to come.

In Chapter 4, we will dive deeper into the science of brain health, exploring how hormones, lifestyle, and even genetics play a role in your cognitive well-being. We will also discuss practical strategies, from nutrition and exercise to stress management and sleep that can help protect your brain and reduce your risk. Your brain is your most precious asset, let us take the steps needed to ensure your mind stays sharp, vibrant, and resilient for life.

CHAPTER 5 OVERVIEW

The Mental Struggle is Real

We have all been there at some point in our lives, feeling anxious, stressed, or even *down*, like the weight of everything is just too much. Mental health is something both men and women struggle with, but as women, we often experience it differently. Many women who seek professional help for symptoms of fatigue, headaches, or pain, are brushed off with phrases like "just stress" or "it is all in your head." Our mental health is deeply connected to our physical health, and addressing the root cause is critical to our well-being.

The factors impacting our mental health as women are deeply connected to the everyday realities so many of us face, whether we are balancing a demanding job, managing a household, or often, doing both. Hormonal changes during our menstrual cycle, pregnancy, or menopause can throw our emotions into overdrive, making us feel irritable, anxious, or simply not like ourselves. And let us not forget the invisible weight of societal expectations, the pressure to be the perfect employee, the perfect mom, the perfect partner, and still have dinner on the table. It can be exhausting, and it is no surprise that stress builds up.

But here's what happens: instead of addressing it, we often push through, internalizing that stress until it starts showing up in our bodies. Maybe it is suffering from chronic constipation or acid reflux, nights spent staring at the ceiling because sleep won't come, or that nagging neck pain that just won't go away.

What we often miss is that these physical symptoms are messengers, telling us something deeper needs care.

When we begin to recognize these patterns and understand how deeply intertwined our mental and physical health are, we can start making small, meaningful changes to feel better. It is not about being perfect, it is about giving ourselves the same care and attention we so freely give to everyone else.

By understanding how our bodies respond uniquely to stress and the environment, we can work with our natural strengths instead of fighting against them. This means recognizing when stress is more than just "in your head" and taking steps to address it holistically. In Chapter 5, I will share practical strategies, from mindfulness and movement to nutrition and sleep, which can help you reclaim your mental well-being. Together, we will explore how to build resilience, manage stress, and create a life that supports your mental health. Because when you feel your best, you can live your best.

CHAPTER 6 OVERVIEW

The Balancing Act of Women's Immunity and Autoimmunity

As women, our immune systems are both a source of incredible strength and, at times, a unique challenge. On the one hand, we are better equipped than men to fight off infections, thanks to our robust immune responses. On the other hand, this same strength makes us more susceptible to autoimmune diseases, where our immune system mistakenly attacks our own tissues. It is a double-edged sword—our bodies are built to protect us, but sometimes that very protection turns inward, leading to conditions like lupus, rheumatoid arthritis, Hashimoto's thyroiditis, or multiple sclerosis.

What is even more frustrating is that many of the symptoms we experience, like fatigue, weight gain, hair loss, brain fog, joint pain, or other unexplained issues, are often dismissed or overlooked. It is not uncommon for women to spend years searching for answers, only to find that the diagnostic criteria and lab values used to identify these conditions have historically been based on men's physiology.

But things are changing, because the more we understand, the more we can advocate for ourselves and find healing.

In Chapter 6, we will dive into immunity discussing practical strategies to strengthen your immune system, reduce your risk of autoimmune conditions, and address any imbalances you may already be experiencing. Knowledge is power, and understanding these processes will give you the tools to take charge of your immune health, reduce inflammation, and feel your best.

CHAPTER 7 OVERVIEW

Digestion Differs for Women

Have you ever wondered why digestive issues like bloating, constipation, or irregular bowel movements seem to be more common in women than in men? If you have experienced these challenges, you are not alone. Our digestive systems are intricately connected to uniquely female factors, from the ebb and flow of our hormones to the distinct ways our bodies respond to stress, and even the very anatomy of our gastrointestinal tracts. These differences are not just minor variations; they play a significant role in how we experience digestion and gut health.

For example, hormonal fluctuations throughout our menstrual cycle, pregnancy, or menopause can directly impact gut motility, often slowing digestion and an increasing the likelihood of constipation. Additionally, women tend to have longer, and more tortuous colons compared to men, which can further contribute to slower transit times. Our gut microbiome, the community of bacteria that live in our digestive system, also differs from men's, shaped by hormones, diet, and even stress levels. Since stress is processed differently in women, it can impact vagal tone, the nerve activity that helps regulate digestion. When this balance is disrupted, it can lead to bloating, discomfort, or irregular bowel movements.

With all these factors in play, it is essential to understand the full picture when it comes to women's gut health.

In Chapter 7, we will take a deeper dive into the fascinating differences in digestive health between men and women, exploring how our gut reacts differently to stress, hormones, and even anatomy. By understanding these unique factors, we can create a digestive health plan that works with our bodies, helping us feel more balanced and in control.

CHAPTER 8 OVERVIEW

Building Bones and Brawn

Did you know that 1 in 2 women over the age of 50 with osteoporosis will experience a fracture?[14] Even more concerning, the mortality rate within the first year after a hip fracture is as high as 30%.[15] And it is not just our bones we need to think about, up to 30% of women over 60 will experience sarcopenia, the gradual loss of muscle mass and strength, which increases the risk of falls, fractures, and disability as we age. These are not just statistics; they are realities that many of us will face, and they underscore how important it is to take care of our bones and muscles now.

Mitochondrial health, hormones, chronic inflammation, gut health, and lifestyle factors like stress, diet, and physical activity also play a significant role in shaping our musculoskeletal health. Because our bodies are different, we need a different approach, one that is tailored to our needs as women.

In Chapter 8, I will guide you through the factors that influence your bone and muscle health and help you create a plan that works for you. We will explore how mitochondrial health and hormones like estrogen impact bone density, how gut health affects nutrient absorption, and how stress and inflammation can quietly undermine your strength. I will also share practical strategies, from nutrition and exercise to stress management, to help you build a foundation of resilience and vitality.

As we prepare to move from education to real-life application, I want to invite you into the next part of this journey, one that weaves together my real-life experiences and the stories of other women behind the science.

Final Thoughts

As you read the upcoming chapters, I invite you to step into the exam room with me, to listen to the stories of the women I have had the privilege to treat and walk alongside us as we navigate the unique health challenges women face every day. While their names have been changed to protect their privacy, these stories are real, told by women just like you, confronting genuine health issues.

My hope is that through their experiences, struggles, pain, and triumphs, you will feel empowered to advocate for your health in the exam room and collaborate with your doctor to discover solutions tailored to your unique health needs.

Chapter 2

Hormone Health

"If all you have is a hammer, everything looks like a nail."

—**Abraham Maslow**

For decades, doctors have been taught to use the birth control pill as the default "hammer" for nearly every issue affecting women—whether it is PMS, irregular periods, acne, PCOS, or endometriosis. It is often the first and sometimes only solution offered. This approach stems largely from how the pill effectively suppresses ovulation and regulates hormonal fluctuations, offering temporary relief, but without addressing underlying root causes. Sometimes prescribed to young girls in the early teen years and continued for decades with no other recommendations. For some women, the pill does help to alleviate their symptoms. But what if women were offered more than a quick fix? What if we had access to a range of evidence-based, personalized options that truly addressed the root cause? How transformative could healthcare become?

A Patient Story: Ella's Journey

Let me share a story about Ella, a vibrant 28-year-old who came to me struggling with irregular periods, weight gain, acne, facial hair, and hair loss. Her journey with these symptoms began in middle school, and like so many women, she was prescribed birth control pills as the solution. But despite years of the pill, her symptoms persisted. Her annual medical checkups offered no new insights, just another refill. She was frustrated and began exploring an integrative approach. This is when we met.

When we dug deeper, we discovered that her lab results revealed all the signs of polycystic ovarian syndrome (PCOS). For those of you suffering with similar symptoms, Ella had an elevated anti-müllerian hormone (AMH), LH:FSH ratio, fasting insulin, hemoglobin (HbA1c), blood sugar, and testosterone. She also had an elevated inflammation marker called hs-CRP, along with deficiencies in vitamin D and omega-3s.

But what I discovered to be even more impactful on her health was her childhood story. She grew up in the Midwest, raised by a single mom, and was left to take care of her younger brother. She had to be the one that took care of everyone. That high-stress environment taught her to put others' needs ahead of her own. It also taught her to control every aspect of her life, but that constant pressure was taking a toll on her body.

She struggled with her weight, controlled her food intake, and tracked her macros, which led to yo-yo dieting, food restriction, and high-intensity workouts. Her job was demanding, her sleep was poor, and she constantly felt exhausted. Even in her relationship, she managed the needs of her fiancé and his family. It was overwhelming. She shared that her greatest fear was infertility, especially because her mother and grandmother struggled with obesity, early menopause, and fertility challenges. Ella had always dreamed of having children one day, and I wanted to help her achieve her dream.

As a physician who has spent years walking alongside women on their health journeys, I have learned that our childhood experiences often shape our health in ways we do not always recognize. And this connection is rarely talked about in medicine. Doctors are not taught to link childhood trauma, chronic stress, or early life habits with the adult health challenges women face. But science now acknowledges that these experiences leave a lasting imprint on our biology. For women, this can manifest in conditions like polycystic ovarian syndrome, depression, cancer, coronary artery disease, and many other chronic conditions.

Ella's story is not unique, and that is what makes it so important.

Research now confirms what so many women have quietly endured for years: our past experiences, especially in childhood, can shape our biology and long-term health.

Let us take a closer look at how these experiences and stressors, especially from early life, can directly affect our hormones, shaping the way they function throughout adulthood.

How Childhood Experiences Shape Our Health

You might wonder, "How does my past trauma affect my health today?" It is a great question—one that research, like the landmark Adverse Childhood Experiences (ACE) study, helps us answer.[16] This groundbreaking study looked at how your emotional, psychological, and even physical pain experienced in childhood affects your adult health and well-being later in life.

For women, this connection is extremely important. Childhood experiences often influence mental health and physical health, as well as our relationships in adulthood. These early experiences can leave scars, affecting everything from how we respond to stress to our risk of chronic illnesses. Understanding this link is a crucial step toward healing and improving overall health. If you are curious about how your own childhood experiences might be influencing your health today, I have included an ACE Test for you to explore, found in Appendix A. Taking this test can provide valuable insights and help you take proactive steps toward a healthier future.

Cortisol and Hormones

Let us take a closer look at how childhood stress impacts women's health, particularly its effect on several different hormones.

Have you ever noticed your periods becoming irregular during times of stress? Chronic stress from childhood, as seen in Ella's story, can create long-standing hormonal imbalances leading to heavy bleeding, skipped periods, and even infertility into adulthood. Stress can even mess with your blood sugar, leading to insulin resistance and risk of diabetes. It can also suppress thyroid hormone production, leading to weight gain and fatigue.

Maybe you have noticed your sleep is disrupted during times of stress, and the next day you find yourself overeating and binging on tempting foods? This is because stress can interrupt melatonin and disrupt appetite hormones. Chronic stress leads to elevated cortisol levels, which contributes to systemic inflammation. Over time, high cortisol levels can become dysregulated, failing to respond properly to stress and leading to fatigue, exhaustion, anxiety, and depression.

Women's bodies are uniquely sensitive to stress, often reacting more intensely than men's. Stress can manifest in many forms: mental, emotional, physical, or a combination of all three. When combined with factors like working long hours, restrictive eating, intense workouts, poor sleep, difficult relationships, and exposure to environmental toxins, it creates a perfect storm that disrupts the production and function of our hormones. This disruption can lead to a cascade of health issues, including infertility, heavy bleeding, missed periods, PCOS, PMS, and PMDD (Premenstrual Dysphoric Disorder), a severe form of premenstrual syndrome that affects mood, energy, and overall functioning.[17] These conditions highlight the importance of addressing both past experiences and present stressors to restore balance and well-being.

By understanding these connections, we can take meaningful steps to address stress as the root cause and create a foundation for long-term health and resilience.

Let us explore what stress really is, and more importantly, how you can build resilience, calm your system, and support your hormone health in the process.

Building Stress Resilience

What is stress? You may think of stress as dealing with a difficult boss or struggling with financial issues. For most of us, stress is a normal part of life, we cannot avoid it. But here's the thing: the way we get through stress matters more than the actual stress itself. Our mindset, awareness, and habits shape how resilient we become in the face of adversity. We can build stress resilience based on how we perceive and manage it.

Through my studies in mindfulness, I discovered a game-changing tool that can help you navigate even the most difficult situations. The acronym is **STOP**.

- **S = Stop:** When you are faced with a challenging moment or person, the first step is giving yourself permission to stop and check in with yourself.
- **T = Take a deep breath**.
- **O = Observe the emotion**—is it fear, sadness, or anger? What story am I telling myself? What pattern am I falling into: fight, flight, or freeze?
- **P = Proceed with kindness toward yourself**. Ask: What do I need right now, and what steps should I take next?

This simple yet powerful practice can help you regain clarity and move forward with intention and compassion.

Take a moment to pause and reflect:

Did this resonate with you? Are there areas in your life where you can practice the STOP protocol? Maybe it is during a stressful conversation, a sleepless night, or when you are feeling overwhelmed by all the roles you are expected to juggle. Wherever you are on your journey, remember, grace and awareness go hand in hand.

Finding our breath, reconnecting with our bodies, and tuning into our thoughts and feelings can help us navigate even the toughest times. These practices not only support our emotional well-being but also help balance our network of hormones, allowing us to thrive even through life's storms. By prioritizing self-awareness and self-care, we create resilience and harmony within ourselves, even when external pressures feel overwhelming.

However, it is important to recognize that some stressors, especially those rooted in past trauma or deeply ingrained patterns, may require professional support. Seeking help from a therapist, counselor, or mental health professional can provide valuable tools and insights to address underlying issues and build lasting resilience. Reaching out for help is a courageous step toward healing and growth.

Insulin and Hormones

In addition to cortisol, insulin can also play a significant role in creating imbalances in our hormones, which directly impacts our overall health. Insulin is a hormone that acts like a key, unlocking our cells to absorb blood sugar from the bloodstream. When our cells are inflamed and struggle to absorb blood sugar, insulin levels rise to compensate. This high-insulin state can lead to weight gain and increase our risk for diabetes.

But insulin's impact does not stop there. High insulin also causes inflammation, particularly in our reproductive organs. This inflammation can cause male hormones like testosterone and DHEA (dehydroepiandrosterone) to rise. **These androgens can lead to facial hair growth, acne, hair loss on the scalp, irregular menstrual cycles, and even difficulty with ovulation.**[18] These symptoms are common in conditions like PCOS, which you read about in Ella's story. Now, it is easier to see how conditions like PCOS and infertility are frequently tied to insulin resistance and higher levels of these male hormones.

Here's where things become even more connected. Increased levels of cortisol and insulin contribute to the buildup of belly fat in the abdominal area. This type of fat is more than just extra weight, it functions like an active organ, releasing and regulating hormones that influence appetite, fat storage, inflammation, and overall metabolism. This sets off a vicious cycle of elevated insulin and cortisol, each reinforcing the other and pushing hormone levels further out of balance.

Let us connect the dots: Can you now see how a prescription for birth control pills for Ella was *not* addressing the root cause? Her years of chronic stress and poor sleep had not only disrupted her cortisol levels but also contributed to insulin resistance, which further exacerbated her hormonal imbalances. Her irregular cycles and symptoms of PCOS were a direct reflection of this hormonal cascade.

The good news is that there are ways to restore balance. By addressing elevated blood sugars, managing cortisol levels, promoting weight loss, and reducing inflammation, whether through medications, supplements, or lifestyle changes, we can support our reproductive system and overall health. Healing begins with understanding, and now you have the insight to start building a more balanced foundation.

Thyroid and Hormones

You might be wondering, how does my thyroid fit into the bigger picture of my health and hormones? Your thyroid is the central hub of your hormonal system, deeply interconnected with cortisol, sex hormones, insulin, and even hunger signals. When your thyroid is out of balance, it can disrupt your entire body.

Elevated cortisol from chronic stress can decrease your thyroid hormone, leaving you fatigued and sluggish. An underactive thyroid can also raise a sex hormone binding protein that binds up estrogen and testosterone, leading to irregular cycles, low libido, or fertility issues. Additionally, thyroid imbalances can affect insulin sensitivity, contributing to blood sugar swings, weight gain, or conditions like PCOS. Notice how the thyroid can impact all your other hormones?

Don't lose heart, while healing your thyroid is a journey, it is possible. Regular testing, tuning into your body, and working with a practitioner can help restore balance. By addressing the root causes, you can reclaim your energy, mood, and overall vitality.

Toxins and Hormones

Now that we have seen how your hormones work together, let us talk about environmental toxins. Do they disrupt your balance? Absolutely, and here's how.

There are thousands of hormone **doppelgängers**, also known as endocrine disruptors, found in the products we use every day. Did you know that the BPA in plastic bottles, chemicals in your cosmetics, body care products, the pesticides sprayed on your food, and the Teflon on your non-stick pan all look like estrogen and they can affect your hormones? These toxins can trick your cells into overreacting. Others block real hormones from working or mess with their production, throwing your entire hormonal system off balance.

Toxins can make you gain weight, cause infertility, increase your risk for cancers like breast and ovarian. They can interfere with your insulin signaling, increasing the risk of diabetes and disrupting thyroid hormone production. Toxins can also weaken the immune system and cause chronic inflammation, which may affect your heart, joints, bone density, and mental health. These chemicals disrupt reproductive health by interfering with the normal production, function, and signaling of estrogen, progesterone, and testosterone in the body, leading to irregular menstrual cycles and fertility challenges.

The liver, your body's detox powerhouse, plays a big role in removal of chemicals, toxins, and hormones. Unfortunately, increased belly fat, excessive medications, alcohol, and substances can impair the liver's ability to do its job, clearing these toxins, which leads to buildup and increases the risk of disease.

Here are a few practical steps you can take today to reduce your exposure to these hormone-disrupting toxins.

- Try substituting your plastic containers and bottles with glass or stainless steel.
- Choose organic produce whenever possible and always read ingredient labels.
- Filter your drinking water with a high-quality filtration system.
- Support your liver with detoxifying foods and limit alcohol and processed foods.

Endocrine disruptors are everywhere, but small changes can make a big difference. Use apps like *Think Dirty* (thinkdirtyapp.com) or *Yuka* (yuka.io), and resources like EWG.org to help you find safer alternatives. It is not about perfection; it is about progress. Every step toward a cleaner environment supports your hormonal health.

The Power of Integrative Medicine

By looking at Ella's health through a comprehensive lens, we were able to address not just her hormonal imbalances but also the root causes: her metabolic health, inflammation, stress, mindset, and even the way her past was shaping her present. We started by tackling her insulin resistance, using a continuous glucose monitor to track her sugar levels, and incorporating medication to help stabilize her blood sugar. Ella began to rebuild her relationship with food, focusing on nourishment rather than restriction. Together, we created healthy meal plans, a gentler workout routine, and a consistent bedtime routine. She also dedicated time to exploring her stress responses at home and work, learning to calm her nervous system and improve her gut health.

This is the heart of integrative medicine, an approach that blends the best of conventional medicine with evidence-based lifestyle, nutritional, and emotional therapies to treat the whole person, not just isolated symptoms. It is not about rejecting modern science, but enhancing it by addressing root causes, from cellular imbalances to unresolved stress, so the body can heal deeply.

Ella's journey was not just physical, but it was emotional. Through regular counseling, she processed past wounds that had silently shaped her health. Slowly, her symptoms eased, her cycles stabilized, and she rediscovered balance, culminating in the joyful news of her pregnancy. Her story is a testament to the power of integrative medicine, a reminder that true healing happens when we address the whole person, not just the symptoms.

The Transition Through Menopause

Another topic that takes center stage in women's health is menopause. At some point in our lives, we will all transition into menopause, a time when our estrogen and progesterone levels drop, and our menstrual cycles come to an end. This phase brings profound changes that go far beyond reproduction. Yet, the medical industry has largely failed women in addressing this transition and the myriad of challenges that come with it.

Let us look at another patient of mine, Laura, whose experience reveals just how misunderstood and overlooked this season of life can be, and how the right support can lead to powerful transformation.

A Patient Story: Laura's Journey

Laura, a 50-year-old patient, came to me feeling completely overwhelmed. She was struggling with her mood, often irritable at work and at home, which had led to frequent arguments with her husband. She found it hard to concentrate on her job and couldn't stand her boss. She was deeply frustrated by her stubborn belly fat but admitted to giving in to sugar cravings to combat her late-afternoon fatigue. Her relationship with her husband had become distant, more like roommates than partners, as she had lost all interest in intimacy. She had been told this was just a "normal part of aging" and that she was "just stressed." Antidepressants were offered, but they were not the solution she was looking for.

What Laura shared next is something I hear from so many women. Though she was coming to me at 50, her symptoms began in her mid-30s, with subtle changes she couldn't ignore: stubborn belly fat, shifts in her energy levels, and a growing frustration that her body no longer felt like her own. By her 40s, she was battling mid-afternoon energy crashes, relying on sugary snacks to push through the day. Evenings left her exhausted, slumped on the couch with her laptop, binge-watching shows she could barely recall the next morning. Night after night, she sacrificed sleep, knowing it was not helping but feeling too stuck to break the cycle. This is where, as an integrative doctor, I was able to help Laura reclaim her health and her life.

Maybe you have experienced similar symptoms as Laura and found your doctor had little to offer. Be rest assured, as the medical community continues to learn more about menopause and hormones, we doctors are changing how we approach this transition. Laura's story, like Ella's, is a powerful reminder that you do not have to accept "just aging" as the answer. With the right support, understanding, and tools, you can navigate this phase with grace and rediscover your vitality.

A New Path to Healing

After listening to Laura's story and identifying her symptoms, the next step was clear, we needed a new, more holistic approach that treated her whole self, not just the symptoms. The first step in Laura's healing journey was creating a space where she felt truly heard and understood. So often, women come to me feeling dismissed or overlooked. Most of us can relate and understand that for Laura to begin healing, she needed to feel supported and seen.

We needed to get a clear picture of her hormone levels. Often, women are discouraged from checking their hormone levels because they can vary throughout the month. However, checking hormones during the first and last part of their cycle can give us a helpful snapshot of where they are compared to expected normal values. We started by taking a close look at her hormones, FSH, LH, three forms of estradiol, progesterone, pregnenolone, DHEA-S, testosterone, a full thyroid panel, fasting insulin, HbA1c, and timed salivary cortisol levels, all pieces of the puzzle that helped us understand what was happening in her body.

Based on her symptoms and her age, we discussed her options with hormone replacement therapy. She decided to take prescription bioidentical hormones along with supplements and lifestyle changes. We built a daily routine designed to nourish her from the inside out. We worked on creating a schedule so she could wake up and go to bed at the same time every day, even on weekends, to balance her circadian rhythms. Her first act in the morning was to drink water, meditate, and get fifteen minutes of morning sun. We discussed the importance of eating within an hour of rising and focusing on regular high-protein meals to keep her energy steady. We shifted her workouts from intense cardio to resistance training to strengthen both her body and her confidence. We also layered in a daily walking program, which became a cherished time for her to move her body and clear her mind.

Laura made some powerful lifestyle changes, too, cutting out alcohol, caffeine, and refined sugar, and creating a calming bedtime ritual that included shutting off all technology an hour before bed. She purchased an Oura ring, a sleep tracker, to create awareness around the habits that were sabotaging her sleep. To support her sleep even further, she decided to try magnesium and ashwagandha, an adaptogenic herb known for its ability to support stress response and promote relaxation, which made a noticeable difference in helping her feel more rested and balanced.[19]

With regular coaching and ongoing support, Laura began to see shifts, not just in her lab results, but in how she felt every day. Her mood brightened, her energy improved, and those small, consistent changes started to add up. Most importantly, Laura regained a sense of control over her health. She no longer felt like her body was working against her; instead, she felt empowered, knowing she had the tools and support to thrive.

Hormones and Women's Health: What You Need to Know

Laura's story is just one of thousands. What she experienced, the confusion, exhaustion, dismissal, is far too common for women navigating hormonal changes.

Here's the thing, doctors are not taught in medical school that women can start their transition into menopause as early as their mid-thirties. Even if your periods seem "normal," your estrogen, progesterone, testosterone, cortisol, and other hormones may already be fluctuating. But because these changes happen gradually, they often go unnoticed, or worse, dismissed.

At times, you may feel utterly drained, battling mood swings, weight that will not budge, sleepless nights, thinning hair, and a libido that has disappeared. You know something is not right, but when you reach out for help, you are often met with dismissive comments like, "This is just part of being a woman," or "It's all in your head." These early signs of hormonal shifts are frequently overlooked by the medical community, leaving women to struggle in silence, wondering if they are imagining it all.

Many women feel misdiagnosed, ignored, or even gaslit into believing their symptoms are just stress or anxiety. They are told to work out more and eat less, or they are offered medications to address their mood, as if their very real, very physical symptoms are purely psychological. This pattern continues for years, often until they finally stop menstruating and enter menopause. By then, they are desperate for answers, only to be told, "There's nothing we can do."

To make matters worse, many doctors refuse to prescribe hormone therapy because they were taught it is too risky, citing outdated fears about breast cancer, heart attacks, and strokes.

The Truth About Hormone Therapy

So where did all this fear around hormone therapy begin and is it actually justified? Let us take a closer look at the science.

The fear surrounding hormone therapy largely stems from the Women's Health Initiative (WHI) study in the early 2000s, which initially reported increased risks of breast cancer and cardiovascular events.[20] However, what you were not told was that these findings were widely misinterpreted and sensationalized. The women in the study were, on average, in their 60s and 70s, many of whom already had significant health issues. As a result, the data did not apply to younger women entering menopause or to the safer, hormone therapies available today.[21]

Thankfully, we now have better evidence. Research shows that starting hormone replacement therapy (HRT) within the first 10 years of menopause, often called the "window of opportunity", not only alleviates symptoms like hot flashes, night sweats, and mood swings, but also offers significant health benefits. It can reduce the risk of heart disease, osteoporosis, and genitourinary issues.[22] The WHI's estrogen-only arm revealed that women who had hysterectomies and used estrogen alone saw a 22% reduction in breast cancer risk.[23]

You will be happy to know that the benefits of estrogen and progesterone go far beyond treating symptoms. These hormones support brain health and memory, improve heart health by enhancing blood vessel elasticity, lower cholesterol and blood pressure, and combat inflammation. They can also improve sleep, regulate body temperature, boost gut health, and even enhance the microbiome. Additionally, they increase energy, lift mood, reignite libido, prevent UTIs, ease vaginal dryness, reduce body fat, strengthen bones, regulate blood sugar, protect joints, and improve skin health. Imagine feeling energetic, vibrant and healthy again!

Since the WHI study, we have learned that micronized progesterone is safer than the synthetic progesterone used in the research.[24] Transdermal or topical estrogen is now the preferred method of delivery, as it bypasses the liver and is considered safer than oral estrogen.[25] Newer studies confirm that when HRT is personalized and started early in menopause, the benefits far outweigh the risks for most women. For example, a 2017 review in *The Lancet* found that HRT initiated in women under 60 or within 10 years of menopause onset significantly reduced mortality and improved quality of life.[26]

Despite this evidence, many women are still denied access to hormone therapy due to outdated fears. This needs to change. Women deserve to have their symptoms taken seriously and to be offered safe, effective treatments that allow them to thrive during menopause and beyond. If you are considering HRT, have a conversation with your doctor. They can assess your unique medical history and help you weigh the risks and benefits to determine what's best for you.

Nutrition and Menopause

While hormone therapy can be incredibly effective, it is not the only tool available. What you eat also plays a powerful role in how you feel during menopause.

As an integrative doctor, I always emphasize the power of food as medicine, especially during menopause. Many women are unaware that dietary changes can significantly alleviate menopausal symptoms. For instance, the WAVS trial demonstrated that a low-fat, vegan diet, including just ½ cup (86g) of cooked soybeans daily, reduced moderate to severe hot flashes by an impressive 87%.[27] Yet most women are never informed by their doctors that something as simple as adjusting their diet could provide such relief.

Beyond hot flashes, the right dietary choices can help stabilize blood sugar, reduce inflammation, promote weight loss, and support hormonal balance. To achieve this, it is important to minimize processed foods, refined flour and sugar, caffeine, and alcohol. Instead, focus on incorporating nutrient-dense, whole foods into your diet.

Here are six key dietary strategies for menopausal women:

1. **Prioritize Protein:** Aim for 1.0-1.2 grams of protein per kilogram of body weight daily. Adequate protein intake supports bone and muscle health, which is especially important after menopause when the risk of osteoporosis increases. Include lean sources like beans, lentils, tofu, tempeh, fish, and poultry.
2. **Support Liver Health:** The liver plays a crucial role in detoxification and hormone metabolism. Boost its function with cruciferous vegetables (like broccoli, cauliflower, and Brussels sprouts), dark leafy greens, sulfur-rich foods (such as onions

and garlic), and antioxidant-packed fruits and vegetables. Think of colorful greens, berries, carrots, and bell peppers.
3. **Incorporate Phytoestrogens:** Plant-based phytoestrogens, found in foods like soy, flaxseeds, sesame seeds, and yams, can help balance hormones and alleviate menopausal symptoms. These compounds mimic estrogen in the body, providing gentle support during this transitional phase.
4. **Add Omega-3 Fatty Acids:** Omega-3s, found in fatty fish (like salmon and sardines), walnuts, chia seeds, and flaxseeds, are essential for reducing inflammation, supporting brain health, and promoting heart health. They can also help with mood swings and joint pain, which are common during menopause.
5. **Focus on High Fiber Foods:** Build your high-fiber meals around whole grains, legumes, nuts, seeds, fruits, and vegetables. These foods provide essential nutrients, fiber, and antioxidants that support overall health and help manage weight. They support the microbiome that helps with hormone regulation.
6. **Stay Hydrated:** Proper hydration is key to managing symptoms like dry skin and constipation. Aim for plenty of water throughout the day and consider herbal teas like chamomile or peppermint for added benefits.

By following these dietary guidelines, women can not only manage menopausal symptoms like hot flashes but also improve energy levels, support bone health, and reduce the risk of cardiovascular issues, all of which are critical during this phase of life.

Exercise and Menopause

Just as nutrition fuels your body from within, movement helps you channel that energy outward. In the exam room, I cannot overstate the power of exercise during menopause. It is one of the most effective tools for managing symptoms and enhancing overall health during this transformative phase. Regular physical activity helps with weight gain (especially around the belly), strengthens your body, calms your mind, and lifts your spirit. Whether through strength training, cardio, mindful movement, or bursts of intensity, exercise is key to thriving during menopause.

Top Seven Recommendations:

1. **Strength Training (3-4 times/week):** Maintains muscle mass and bone density, reducing osteoporosis risk. Use weights, resistance bands, or bodyweight exercises like squats and lunges.
2. **Cardio (30 minutes daily):** Supports heart health, boosts mood, and improves energy. Some excellent choices are walking, swimming, cycling, or dancing.
3. **HIIT or Sprints (1-2 times/week):** Boosts metabolism, burns fat, and improves cardiovascular fitness. Examples: 20-30 seconds of sprinting or burpees followed by 1-2 minutes of rest.
4. **Time in Nature:** Walk, hike, or garden to combine exercise with nature's healing power.
5. **Mind-Body Practices (Yoga, Pilates, Tai Chi):** Alleviate hot flashes, improve sleep, and promote relaxation while enhancing flexibility and balance.
6. **Endorphin-Boosting Activities:** Exercise releases endorphins, easing mood swings, anxiety, and depression.
7. **Consistency Over Intensity:** Focus on regular, sustainable movement. Small, daily efforts yield significant benefits.

Sleep and Menopause

While movement energizes and strengthens the body, restorative sleep is what allows it to heal and reset. Nearly every menopausal woman I meet shares concerns about sleep, whether it is trouble falling asleep, staying asleep, or waking up at 2 AM to watch the clock. Many describe tossing the covers off and on as their body temperature fluctuates from hot to cold, while others struggle with a racing mind that just won't shut off. Since estrogen plays a key role in regulating body temperature and the brain's sleep centers, hormonal shifts during menopause often disrupt deep, restful sleep. For those who are candidates, hormone replacement therapy (HRT) can be a game-changer for restoring sleep quality.

Five Tips for Better Sleep:

1. **Avoid Blue Light:** Limit exposure to screens in the evening, especially in the hour before bed, to protect melatonin production.
2. **Balance Blood Sugar:** Include a complex carb at dinner to stabilize blood sugar through the night.
3. **Limit Alcohol:** While it may seem relaxing, alcohol disrupts sleep and mood and is linked to an increased risk of breast cancer. Aim for less than two servings per week or eliminate it.
4. **Create a Sleep-Friendly Environment:** Keep your bedroom cool, dark, and quiet, and reserve it solely for sleep and intimacy.
5. **Natural Remedies:** Some women find relief with sleepy time teas, magnesium, GABA, L-theanine, ashwagandha, or inositol. Always consult your doctor before trying supplements to ensure they are safe and appropriate for you.

Small, consistent changes can make a big difference in helping you reclaim restful, restorative sleep during menopause.

Suggested Supplements for Hormone Health

Hormone health is essential for overall well-being, influencing everything from energy levels and mood to metabolism and reproductive health. While quality sleep is a critical piece of the puzzle, it's just one part of a bigger picture. Nutrition, movement, emotional well-being, and targeted supplementation can also offer powerful support, especially during times of hormonal change.

Certain well-researched supplements have been shown to help maintain hormonal balance. However, lifestyle factors like diet, exercise, and stress management remain foundational. Always consult your healthcare provider before starting any new supplement, particularly if you have a medical condition or are taking medications. For a list of evidence-based supplements that may support hormone health, see **Appendix B**.

Final Thoughts

The stories of Ella and Laura highlight the need for a shift in how we approach women's health, one that prioritizes root causes, personalized care, and empowerment. By understanding the interconnectedness of our hormones, stress, and lifestyle, we can envision a future where women no longer feel dismissed or overlooked, but are instead supported in achieving lasting, vibrant health.

Your health is more than just a set of symptoms to manage, it reflects your whole story. And as women, we deserve care that honors that story, care that sees us as more than just a diagnosis.

Questions to Discuss With Your Doctor:

These questions are designed to help you have a more informed, collaborative conversation with your healthcare provider, so you can get to the root of what's going on and build a plan that supports your mental, emotional, and physical well-being.

1. Can I get a full hormone panel to assess my hormone levels?

Consider: Sex hormones like estrogen, progesterone, and testosterone, tested in both the follicular and luteal phases if menstruating, AMH (if applicable), fasting insulin, HbA1c, blood sugars, full thyroid panel (TSH, free T3, free T4, reverse T3, thyroid antibodies), timed salivary cortisol, leptin, comprehensive lipids, and inflammatory markers like hs-CRP and uric acid.

2. Am I a candidate for hormone replacement therapy (HRT)?

Discuss: The risks, benefits, and alternatives to HRT based on your symptoms, health history, and lab results.

3. Are there any supplements or natural therapies that can help balance my hormones?

Consider: Adaptogenic herbs like ashwagandha or rhodiola, vitamin D, omega-3 fatty acids, magnesium, and targeted nutrients like DIM or Vitex for hormone support.

> **4. Are there dietary changes that could support my hormone balance?**

Discuss: Anti-inflammatory diets, blood sugar-balancing strategies, or specific nutrients to support hormone production and metabolism.

> **5. What can I do to manage stress and improve sleep, as these impact hormone health?**

Consider: Stress management techniques like meditation, yoga, or deep breathing, and sleep hygiene practices to support restorative sleep.

> **6. Can you refer me to specialists who can help me further?**

Consider: A menopause expert, a nutritionist for personalized dietary guidance, a psychologist for stress or mood support, an exercise trainer for tailored fitness plans, or a yoga instructor for stress reduction and flexibility.

> **7. Can we partner together to create a preventative health plan for hormone balance?**

Work with your doctor to develop a personalized plan that addresses your unique needs, symptoms, and goals.

For a complete companion resource, including all "Questions to Discuss with Your Doctor," Supplement Lists, and Guides, scan the QR code.

Chapter 3

Heart Health

"The human heart is the engine of life."

—Leonardo da Vinci

As a South Asian woman, heart disease runs deep in my family. All the men in my family have heart disease—my maternal grandfather, three uncles and even my husband all struggle with high cholesterol, diabetes, and heart disease. But what truly hit home was to find out my mom also had heart disease. She didn't have the typical risk factors, yet she was diagnosed and needed a stent in her coronary artery. Her symptom? Back pain. Not the classic chest pain we so often associate with heart disease. It was a wake-up call for me.

Despite being a physician, I realized how deeply ingrained the bias is that heart disease is a "man's disease," presenting as someone clutching their chest. My mom's experience opened my eyes to the reality that women's heart health is often overlooked, even by those of us in the medical field. It was a moment that changed how I view heart disease and reinforced the importance of listening to the unique ways it can manifest in women.

My mom's story was a wake-up call for me, and I hope this chapter serves as one for you. You deserve to feel empowered, informed, and in control of your heart health, because your heart matters, and so do you. And while my mom's experience felt like an exception, the truth is, it is far more common than we think.

How Women's Heart Disease Presents Differently

Heart disease in women often goes unrecognized because its symptoms can look very different from what we typically associate with heart attacks. While both men and women can experience the classic "crushing chest pain," we as women are more likely to have symptoms that are subtle and easily brushed off as something else. Fatigue, nausea, shortness of breath, jaw pain, abdominal discomfort, or even back pain, like what my own mother experienced, can all be signs of a heart attack. Too often, these symptoms are dismissed as stress, anxiety, indigestion, or just a normal part of aging. But this misunderstanding can lead to delays in seeking care, or even misdiagnoses, putting us at greater risk.

What's more, women are more likely to experience what is called a "silent" heart attack, where symptoms are so mild or unusual that they go unnoticed. This is especially dangerous because it means damage to the heart can happen without us even realizing it, increasing our risk of more severe cardiac events in the future.

But there is hope. The good news is that heart disease is largely preventable, and knowledge is your greatest tool. As you continue reading, you will learn about the warning signs, risk factors and prevention, all geared toward positioning you as your own best advocate, taking control of your heart health.

Symptoms to Not Ignore:

To help you better understand the signs, here are some of the most common, but often overlooked, symptoms of heart disease in women.

- **Fatigue:** Unusual or extreme tiredness that does not improve with rest.
- **Abdominal pain, nausea, or vomiting:** Sometimes mistaken for indigestion.
- **Shortness of breath:** Difficulty breathing, especially when it happens without exertion.
- **Pain in other areas:** Discomfort in one or both arms, the back, neck, jaw, or stomach.
- **Chest pain or pressure:** While not always present, this can still occur and may feel like tightness, squeezing, or fullness that lasts more than a few minutes or comes and goes.
- **Lightheadedness or dizziness:** Feeling sick to your stomach or dizzy, which may be mistaken for the flu or low blood sugar.
- **Cold sweat:** Breaking out in a cold sweat for no apparent reason.

The fact is, heart disease is the leading cause of death for women, yet it is underdiagnosed, undertreated, and misunderstood. Over 60 million women (44%) in the U.S. are living with some form of heart disease, leading to 1 in every 5 female deaths.[28]

Women are more likely than men to be told their symptoms are due to anxiety, stress, or aging. This bias does not just exist in healthcare settings, it is systemic. Only about half of all women (56%) recognize that heart disease is their number one killer. That lack of awareness can have deadly consequences.[29] So let us break it down. In the next section, we will explore exactly why heart disease shows up differently in women and what makes it so often missed.

A Patient Story: Maggie's Journey – How Women's Heart Disease Develops Differently

Let me share a story about one of my dearest friends, Maggie. We met on the first day of medical school. Though we were a few years apart in age and couldn't have been more different, something magical brought us together, and we became thick as thieves during that first year. She was athletic and loved sports, while I was fearful of any social activities involving sports and had no idea about professional teams, players, or upcoming bowls. Yet, despite our differences, we clicked right away.

We were initially paired together in the first block of classes, and then we chose to team up for the next three blocks. Together, we became a force to be reckoned with in our medical class. Maggie was smart, direct, decisive, confident, and funny. We spent countless hours studying for our medical boards and shared every Thursday night meal for four years, watching the newest episodes of *Friends* and *ER* with enthusiasm and ritual. Those shows became our tradition, a comforting constant during the toughest years of our lives. We leaned on each other, and it was our friendship and unbreakable bond that got us through.

After graduation, we chose our respective specialties and parted ways. But over the years, we stayed in touch, playing significant roles in each other's lives through marriages, children, relocations, job changes, moments of joy, and times of grief. Our connection remained strong, no matter the distance or life's twists and turns.

Then, one day, Maggie called me with a health concern. She had undergone a screening coronary artery calcium (CAC) score test and was told her score was 1200. For those unfamiliar, it is a CAT scan of your heart arteries and a score over 400 is considered very high, indicating significant calcium buildup and a very elevated risk of heart disease.

What made this even more shocking was that Maggie had no standard risk factors. She was not overweight, didn't smoke, stayed physically active, was not diabetic, had normal blood pressure, and had no symptoms. After finding significant calcified plaque on a heart scan, her doctor placed her on a statin, and nothing more was offered to reduce her risk of a future heart attack or stroke. And no further investigation into her risk factors was performed. After menopause, she was not offered hormone therapy because her physician at the time was concerned about the potential associated risk of breast cancer.

How did this happen to Maggie? I am sure as you are reading, you are wondering if this can happen to you. Maggie's story highlights how even the most seemingly healthy among us can face unexpected health challenges. It also raises important questions about the pathophysiology of heart disease in women. Why do women like Maggie, with no traditional risk factors, still develop significant coronary artery disease? What role do hormones, inflammation, or microvascular dysfunction play in women's heart health? And why are these factors so often overlooked in conventional medical approaches?

These are the very questions that demand a closer look. To truly understand why women like Maggie develop heart disease, often without the typical risk factors, we need to explore the unique ways it manifests in the female body. Let us examine the hidden physiological differences that make heart disease in women so often misunderstood and misdiagnosed.

Four Hidden Heart Risks: Why Women's Heart Disease is So Often Missed

Maggie's story is not an isolated one and it underscores a larger issue: heart disease often looks different in women, which is why it is so frequently misdiagnosed or missed altogether. As discussed, heart disease develops differently in women. Our hearts are smaller, more prone to inflammation, tied to our hormones, and when sick, do not act like men's hearts. They respond less to standard treatments and often have poorer outcomes.

1. Smaller Arteries, Bigger Challenges

For starters, women tend to have smaller coronary arteries than men. This might seem like a minor detail, but it is a big deal when it comes to blood flow. Smaller arteries mean less room for blood to move freely, especially when plaque starts to build up. And speaking of plaque, here's where things get even more interesting.

In men, plaque often forms as large, localized blockages that are easier to spot on standard tests like angiograms. But in women, plaque tends to spread more evenly along the artery walls, a condition called diffuse scattered erosive plaque. This makes it much harder to detect using traditional diagnostic tools, which are designed to catch those big, obvious blockages. As a result, women are often told their arteries look "clear," even when they are not.

From these physical differences in artery structure, we move into another often-missed condition that impacts women more frequently:

2. The Hidden Threat: Coronary Microvascular Disease

Another reason heart disease flies under the radar in women is coronary microvascular disease (MVD). This condition affects the tiny arteries in the heart, which do not show up on standard tests. Women with MVD often experience chest pain, fatigue, and shortness of breath, even when their larger arteries appear perfectly healthy. It is like having a hidden fire smoldering beneath the surface, one that does not show up on the radar until it is too late.

In addition to these small vessel issues, the lining of our blood vessels plays a role that is often overlooked:

3. Endothelial Dysfunction: The Silent Saboteur

Now, let us talk about the endothelium, the delicate inner lining of your blood vessels. Think of the endothelium as the Teflon coating on a nonstick pan, keeping everything in the blood vessel gliding effortlessly. In a healthy state, the endothelium produces nitric oxide, a molecule that helps blood vessels relax and stay flexible. But after menopause, the blood vessels can become stiff and inflamed, like a garden hose left in the sun, dry, cracked, and less flexible.

The loss of estrogen is a major culprit. Estrogen protects the endothelium by reducing inflammation and oxidative stress. When estrogen levels drop, nitric oxide production decreases, and the endothelium becomes eroded and more prone to plaque buildup (atherosclerosis) or, in some women, a sudden tear in the artery wall (called SCAD) where the layers separate like peeling wallpaper. This can lead to heart disease and high blood pressure, even without obvious blockages. It is like the Teflon coating wearing off, causing everything to stick and making it harder for blood to flow smoothly.

One more hidden contributor to women's heart disease is often missed until it becomes a major threat:

4. Arterial Calcifications: The Hidden Danger

Another piece of the puzzle is calcium deposits that form in the walls of your arteries (arterial calcifications), like in Maggie's case. These calcifications are often a response to chronic inflammation, injury, or stress, and they are more common in women than many realize. In women, these deposits can be more diffuse and harder to detect, yet they significantly increase the risk of heart attacks and strokes.

The loss of estrogen after menopause accelerates this process. Estrogen acts as a natural shield against inflammation and oxidative stress, both of which contribute to endothelial injury and calcification. But it is not just estrogen loss. Factors like chronic stress, environmental toxins, inflammatory conditions (such as lupus or rheumatoid arthritis), high blood pressure, high blood sugar, and elevated cholesterol also fuel this dangerous buildup. Without estrogen's protection, and with these additional triggers, the risk of calcifications skyrockets, further complicating the picture of heart disease in women.

Why Women Are Diagnosed Later

These biological differences mean that women are often diagnosed with heart disease later than men, when the disease is more advanced and harder to treat. Standard diagnostic tools and treatment protocols were largely developed based on research in men, leaving women at a disadvantage. It is why stories like Maggie's are so important, they highlight the urgent need for a deeper understanding of how heart disease manifests in women and why we must advocate for more personalized, proactive approaches to prevention and treatment.

So, if women are at higher risk of delayed diagnosis, what steps can we take to get ahead of the curve?

What Can We Do? Your Heart, Your Power

So, what does this mean for you? First, it is about awareness. Know your risk factors, know your numbers, and listen to your body. If you are experiencing symptoms like chest pain, fatigue, shortness of breath, or even unexplained nausea, do not dismiss them. Advocate for yourself and seek out healthcare providers who understand how heart disease uniquely presents in women.

Second, focus on prevention. Heart disease is largely preventable, and small, consistent changes can make a big difference. I will share more on this later in the chapter.

Your heart is the engine that keeps you going, and it deserves your attention and care. By understanding how heart disease develops uniquely in women, we can take control of our health and rewrite the narrative.

Now let us look more closely at what sets women apart, not just in symptoms but in the very risks we face.

Seven Overlooked Risk Factors That Make Women's Heart Disease Different

Do you know if you are at risk of a heart attack? While women do share some risk factors with men, like high cholesterol, high blood pressure, smoking, diabetes, excess weight, a sedentary lifestyle, poor diet, stress, depression, and alcohol use, they also have unique risk factors that often go overlooked. Shockingly, these are not routinely taught in medical schools, residency programs, or even continued education. I have rarely seen this topic addressed in conferences, exams, or training, which is why I'm sharing this with you now. If any of the following applies to you, do not hesitate to ask your healthcare provider about heart screening. You deserve care, and it starts with the right conversation.

1. Menstruation Issues and Heart Disease

Your menstrual health is deeply tied to your heart health. If you started your period before age 11 or entered menopause before 40, it can increase your risk of high cholesterol, high blood pressure, and inflammation, all of which are risk factors for heart disease. Also, if you have been diagnosed with Polycystic Ovarian Syndrome (PCOS), you are at higher risk for insulin resistance, weight gain, and elevated androgens, which can lead to hypertension, diabetes, and ultimately, heart disease.

2. Autoimmune Diseases and Heart Disease

Autoimmune conditions like lupus and rheumatoid arthritis cause chronic inflammation, which damages blood vessels, increases arterial stiffness, and raises the risk of plaque buildup or rupture. Women make up 80% of autoimmune cases, and if you have one of these conditions, you are 4 to 5 times more likely to develop heart disease.[30] Despite this, women with autoimmune diseases are rarely screened early for heart issues, leaving them vulnerable to preventable complications.

3. Pregnancy Complications

Your pregnancy history can be a crystal ball for future heart disease risk. If you have experienced:
- Pre-term delivery
- Pre-eclampsia
- Diabetes or high blood pressure during pregnancy
- A baby with low or high birth weight

Your risk of heart disease later in life increases significantly. Yet women are rarely asked about pregnancy complications during heart risk assessments. Has your doctor ever brought this up? If not, it is time to start the conversation yourself.

4. Menopause

As we have discussed in Chapter 2, menopause is a game-changer for heart health. Before menopause, estrogen protects your heart, but after menopause, your risk of heart disease skyrockets. Without estrogen, your blood vessels stiffen, inflammation rises, and cholesterol, blood sugar, and blood pressure often follow suit. Menopause can also increase susceptibility to gum disease, which impacts heart health. Talk to your doctor about whether hormone therapy might be right for you, every woman's journey is different, and the right support can make all the difference.

5. Migraines

Did you know migraines, especially those with aura (visual or sensory disturbances), are a significant risk factor for heart disease in women? Research shows they are linked to a higher risk of stroke, heart attacks, and other cardiovascular events. Because migraines share the same issues as heart disease, like inflammation, endothelial dysfunction, and changes in blood vessel behavior. Hormonal fluctuations during perimenopause and menopause can worsen both migraines and increase cardiovascular risk.

6. Hot Flashes

Frequent or severe hot flashes are not just annoying, they are a red flag for heart health. They are linked to endothelial dysfunction, higher blood pressure, and unfavorable cholesterol changes. Hot flashes may be a sign that your cardiovascular system may be under stress. Addressing them through lifestyle changes, hormone therapy, or targeted treatments can improve your quality of life and reduce heart disease risk.

7. Mental Health

Stress, depression, and anxiety can hit women harder and take a toll on your heart. Chronic stress ramps up cortisol, driving inflammation, damaging blood vessels, raising blood pressure, and disrupting cholesterol balance. Women are twice as likely as men to experience stress-related conditions like depression and anxiety, and they are more susceptible to stress-induced heart conditions like Takotsubo cardiomyopathy (broken heart syndrome), which mimics a heart attack.

If you are feeling overwhelmed, anxious, or persistently down, talk to your doctor. Managing stress through lifestyle changes, therapy, or other treatments can protect both your mental and heart health.

How Women's Heart Labs Differ from Men's

If you have had blood work done to look at your risk for heart disease, your doctor may not be looking at the correct lab tests or normal ranges for women. The Framingham Heart Study, one of the most influential long-term studies on cardiovascular health, uncovered critical differences in how heart disease is tested and treated in women versus men.[31] Here's what you need to know about how women's heart labs can tell a different story.

Blood Testing Differences

Did you know women have different "normal" lab ranges than men? Here is what you need to know to accurately assess your heart disease risk:

- **Troponin Levels:** When you go to the ER with chest pain, doctors check your troponin levels to see if you are having a heart attack. But did you know women's levels are often lower than men's and most ER doctors do not know that. They are taught that a troponin level under 0.1 ng/mL is "normal," but women having a heart attack may have levels just above 0.05 ng/mL. This means many women are missed or misdiagnosed because the standard is based on men. Gender-specific thresholds are essential to accurately diagnose and treat women, while a few medical centers across the country have implemented these new lab standards, far more adoption is needed.
- **HDL Cholesterol (Good Cholesterol):** HDL is more protective for women than men. Women typically have higher HDL levels, which is good, but low HDL is a stronger predictor of heart disease risk in women. For women, an HDL level below 50 mg/dL is a risk factor, while for men, it is below 40 mg/dL.
- **LDL Cholesterol (Bad Cholesterol):** High LDL is a risk factor for both men and women, but it is especially harmful for women after menopause. As estrogen declines, LDL levels rise, and HDL drops, increasing heart disease risk.
- **Triglycerides:** High triglycerides are a stronger predictor of heart disease in women than in men. Levels over 150 mg/dL, especially paired with low HDL, significantly increase a woman's risk. Your triglyceride level should be less than twice your HDL.
- **Inflammatory Markers:** Conditions like autoimmune diseases, which are more common in women, can elevate markers like high sensitivity C-reactive protein (hs-CRP), signaling a higher

risk of heart disease. Additional cardiac inflammation markers, lipoprotein analysis, oxidized LDL, uric acid, insulin and HbA1c can help assess your cardiac risk.

Why This Matters

Women's hearts are different, and so are their lab results. Understanding these differences is crucial for accurate diagnosis and treatment. If you are concerned about your heart health, do not hesitate to ask for the right tests and advocate for gender-specific care. Your heart deserves nothing less.

Treatment Differences:

Maybe you have put on a cholesterol lowering medication like a statin. Did you know standard treatments for heart disease, such as statins and stents, were largely developed based on studies conducted on men? As a result, these treatments are often less effective for women. For example:

- **Statins**: Women are more likely to experience side effects from statins, such as muscle pain and liver issues, which can lead to discontinuation of the medication.
- **Aspirin**: The benefits of aspirin for preventing heart attacks are less clear in women, especially younger women. While aspirin can reduce the risk of stroke in women over 65, its protective effect against heart attacks is more pronounced in men.
- **Stents and bypass surgery**: Women tend to have poorer outcomes after these procedures, partly because their arteries are smaller, and plaque is more diffuse.
- **Medication dosing**: Women often require lower doses of certain medications due to differences in body composition, metabolism, and hormone levels.

- **Hormone Replacement Therapy**: HRT can be beneficial for heart health. Starting HRT within the first 10 years of menopause, often referred to as the "window of opportunity", may have protective benefits for the heart. These benefits include improving cholesterol profiles (raising HDL and lowering LDL), reducing inflammation, enhancing blood vessel function, and potentially lowering the risk of heart disease. However, HRT is not a one-size-fits-all solution. It is essential to have a detailed discussion with your doctor to weigh the risks and benefits based on your health profile.
- **Holistic approaches**: Lifestyle changes like a heart-healthy diet, regular exercise, and stress management are shown to be more beneficial in women. Evidence-based supplements should always be discussed with your doctor.

By recognizing these differences, we can move toward more personalized and effective care for women's heart health.

What You Can Do: Prevention and Proactivity

The good news is that heart disease is largely preventable, and knowledge is your greatest tool. Here is how you can take control of your heart health and thrive, especially during pivotal times like menopause:

Know Your Numbers: Regular check-ups are essential for understanding your heart health. Consider these advanced tests for a comprehensive view of your cardiovascular and metabolic health:

Advanced Cholesterol Profile

Traditionally includes Total Cholesterol, LDL, Triglycerides, HDL, and non-HDL cholesterol numbers. Additional advanced tests can provide a more comprehensive view.

- **Apolipoprotein B (Apo B):** Measures the number of atherogenic particles (such as LDL, VLDL, and lipoprotein(a)). Elevated levels, especially in women, can signal higher heart disease risk, even if LDL levels are normal.
- **Lipoprotein Analysis**: Evaluate the size and number of lipid particles, since smaller, denser LDL particles are more likely to cause plaque buildup. Women tend to have a higher proportion of these harmful particles.
- **Lipoprotein(a):** A key marker for heart disease risk, elevated levels of lipoprotein(a) are linked to an increased risk of cardiovascular events, independent of other cholesterol levels.

Genetic Testing for Heart Disease

Some genetic tests can identify inherited conditions that increase the risk of heart disease, such as familial hypercholesterolemia or certain mutations that affect lipid metabolism.

Metabolic Markers: These tests provide insight into your metabolic health, which can affect cardiovascular risk.

- **Fasting Insulin**: Helps assess insulin resistance, a factor in heart disease and metabolic health.
- **HbA1c**: Measures long-term blood sugar control, offering insights into diabetes risk.
- **Uric Acid**: Linked to inflammation and metabolic health and associated with gout and heart disease.

- **Homocysteine Levels**: High levels of homocysteine, an amino acid in the blood, are linked to an increased risk of heart disease. This test helps assess whether elevated homocysteine levels are a contributing factor.
- **Waist-to-Hip Ratio**: A higher ratio can indicate visceral fat, a major risk factor for heart disease. Goal for women <0.8 and men <1.0.

Inflammation Markers

Elevated inflammation levels are linked to a higher risk of cardiovascular disease.
- **High-Sensitivity C-Reactive Protein (hsCRP):** A marker of systemic inflammation, important for assessing heart disease risk.
- **Lp-PLA2 (Lipoprotein-associated Phospholipase A2):** Associated with vascular inflammation and plaque instability. Elevated levels indicate a higher risk of heart attack or stroke.
- **MPO (Myeloperoxidase):** A marker of oxidative stress and inflammation in the arteries, often elevated in women with microvascular dysfunction.
- **ADMA and SDMA:** Reflect endothelial dysfunction and reduced nitric oxide production, which are more common in women, particularly after menopause.

Imaging:

The following imaging tests provide a thorough picture of your health, helping you catch potential issues early before they become serious:
- **Coronary Artery Calcium (CAC) Score**: A CT scan that measures the amount of calcium buildup in your coronary

arteries. A higher CAC score indicates a higher risk of heart disease. It helps assess the presence of early-stage coronary artery disease even before symptoms appear.

- **Carotid Ultrasound**: An imaging test that checks for plaque buildup in the carotid arteries, which supply blood to the brain. This test helps identify early signs of atherosclerosis and stroke risk.
- **Ankle-Brachial Index (ABI):** A simple test that compares the blood pressure in the ankle with the blood pressure in the arm to check for peripheral artery disease (PAD), a condition where narrowed arteries reduce blood flow to the limbs.
- **Echocardiogram**: An ultrasound of the heart that provides detailed images of the heart's structure and function. It can assess heart muscle strength, valve function, and blood flow.
- **Stress Test (Exercise or Pharmacologic):** Measures how your heart responds to physical stress (exercise) or medication-induced stress. This test helps detect blockages in the coronary arteries, arrhythmias, and other heart-related issues.

Listening to Your Body:

If something feels off, whether it is unexplained fatigue, shortness of breath, chest discomfort, or even subtle signs like jaw pain or nausea, do not dismiss it. As you are now aware, your unique symptoms of heart disease are subtle and easier to overlook. Advocate for yourself and insist on further testing if your concerns are not addressed. Remember, you know your body best.

Foods That Decrease Inflammation:

Since heart disease is fundamentally an inflammatory condition in women, the best way to fight inflammation is through your diet. The Mediterranean diet, backed by decades of research, is a gold standard for heart health. It emphasizes whole, nutrient-dense foods like leafy greens, fatty fish (rich in omega-3s), olive oil, nuts, seeds, and antioxidant-packed berries. Studies, such as the PREDIMED trial, have shown that the Mediterranean diet reduces the risk of heart attacks, strokes, and cardiovascular death by up to 30%.[32] It also improves cholesterol levels, reduces blood pressure, and supports healthy blood sugar levels. Aim to fill your plate with colorful, whole foods and minimize processed foods, refined sugars, and trans fats.

Managing Stress:

While stress can be difficult to eliminate completely, chronic stress is a silent contributor to heart disease. It raises cortisol levels, which can lead to high blood pressure, inflammation, and insulin resistance. Work on reducing your stress with a daily routine of mindfulness meditation, yoga, deep breathing exercises, or even journaling. These practices not only calm your nervous system but also improve your emotional resilience, helping you navigate life's challenges with greater ease.

Moving Your Body:

With our busy schedules, regular exercise can be difficult to incorporate. However, it is critical for us to understand that regular exercise is one of the most effective ways to support heart health. Aim for a mix of strength training (to build muscle and boost metabolism) and aerobic activity (like brisk walking, swimming, or cycling) to improve circulation and strengthen your heart. Even small changes, like taking the stairs or walking after meals, can make a big difference. Studies show that just 30 minutes of moderate exercise five times a week can reduce your risk of heart disease by up to 40%.[33]

Ten Suggested Supplements for Heart Health

For heart disease, certain evidence-based supplements have shown clear benefits in supporting heart health. However, it is important to note that supplements should never replace prescribed medications or lifestyle changes. Consult your healthcare provider before starting any new supplement, especially if you have a heart condition or are taking medications. See Appendix B for a list of these recommended supplements for heart health.

Final Thoughts

While women's heart health is complex, it does not have to be confusing. We can rewrite the narrative by understanding how heart disease affects us and begin taking proactive steps to protect our health. My mom's story was a wake-up call for me, and I hope this chapter serves as one for you. You deserve to feel empowered, informed, and in control of your heart health, because your heart matters, and so do you.

Let us stop dismissing women's symptoms and start taking them seriously. Together, we can close the gap in care and ensure that no woman's heart health is overlooked again.

Questions to Discuss With Your Doctor:

These questions are designed to help you have a more informed, collaborative conversation with your healthcare provider, so you can get to the root of what is going on and build a plan that supports your mental, emotional, and physical well-being.

1. Can I get a comprehensive cardiac panel to assess my risk for heart disease?

Consider: Lipid panel (total cholesterol, LDL, HDL, triglycerides), apolipoprotein B (ApoB), lipoprotein(a), hs-CRP, homocysteine, fasting insulin, HbA1c, blood sugars, and inflammatory markers like IL-6 and TNF-alpha. See the above list.)

2. Would advance testing like a coronary calcium score or carotid ultrasound be helpful?

These tests can provide insights into plaque buildup and arterial health, helping to assess your risk of heart disease.

3. How can I reduce inflammation and support my heart through diet?

Discuss: Anti-inflammatory diets like the Mediterranean diet, reducing processed foods and added sugars, and incorporating heart-healthy fats like omega-3s and olive oil.

4. Are there other lifestyle changes you would recommend supporting my heart health?

Consider: Regular exercise, smoking and alcohol cessation, weight management, and strategies to improve sleep quality.

5. Are there any supplements that can help support my heart health?

Consider: Omega-3 fatty acids, CoQ10, magnesium, vitamin D, and antioxidants.

6. What medications or therapies might be appropriate for my heart health?

Discuss: Cholesterol lowering medications, blood pressure medications, or other therapies based on your risk factors and lab results.

7. What can I do to manage stress, as it impacts heart health?

Consider: Stress management techniques like meditation, yoga, deep breathing, or mindfulness practices.

8. Can we evaluate my sleep patterns, as poor sleep can affect heart health?

Discuss: Sleep hygiene practices, testing for sleep apnea, or referrals to a sleep specialist if needed.

> **9. Can you refer me to specialists who can help me further?**

Consider: A nutritionist for personalized dietary guidance, a cardiologist for advanced care, or a stress management coach.

> **10. Can we partner together to create a preventative health plan for my heart?**

Work with your doctor to develop a personalized plan that addresses your unique needs, risk factors, and goals.

For a complete companion resource, including all "Questions to Discuss with Your Doctor," Supplement Lists, and Guides, scan the QR code.

Chapter 4

Brain Health

"Women's brains are not the same as men's brains."

—**Dr. Lisa Mosconi**

When I made rounds visiting my patients at a nursing home in my small Arizona town, I noticed something unusual: the halls were filled with elderly women, with only a handful of men scattered among them. It is no secret that women tend to outlive men by about six years on average.[34] But as I walked through the dementia ward, I saw something even more striking—most of the residents struggling with memory loss were women.

At first glance, you might think, "Well, women live longer, so of course they are more likely to develop Alzheimer's or dementia." And yes, nearly two-thirds of Alzheimer's cases are women, and age is the biggest risk factor. But the story does not end there.[35]

The truth is it is not just about living longer. The reasons behind women's higher risk of dementia are deeper, more intricate, and tied to the unique biology and experiences of the female brain. As women, our longevity advantage is literally woven into our DNA. Those powerful XX chromosomes carry genes that help us combat oxidative stress and aging. They produce enzymes that repair cell damage caused by free radicals, pollution, and toxins, giving us resilience and vitality. Yet, this same biology also makes our brains uniquely vulnerable as we age.

So, what is really happening beneath the surface?

Dementia risk in women is shaped by a complex mix of factors: our genetics, hormones, inflammation levels, stress, environmental exposures, energy production, and even our life experiences. This chapter will take you on a journey through the female brain, a story of resilience, neuroplasticity, and vulnerability. What you are going to learn about is how our brains adapt and remodel themselves over time (the very definition of neuroplasticity).[36]

More importantly, you will learn about the meaningful steps you can take to protect your brain health and thrive for years to come. Because your brain, your incredible, adaptable, powerful brain, deserves nothing less.

A Patient Story: Linda's Journey

Let me tell you about Linda and her health journey. Linda was a 58-year-old woman who came to me after seeing her primary care physician. She had started noticing subtle changes in her memory, forgetting the names of people she recently met, occasionally misplacing her keys, and struggling with focus at work.

She felt frustrated because she was told, *"Your symptoms are a normal part of aging,"* and no further recommendations were made. But Linda was not convinced. Her mother had lived with Alzheimer's disease, and Linda was her primary caregiver for years, watching her slowly deteriorate until she could no longer care for herself. The fear of walking the same path haunted her. That is when we met. Linda was seeking an integrative path to maintaining her brain health so she would not suffer the same fate as her mother.

We started by talking by taking a thorough look at her medical history, lifestyle, work, relationships, diet, stress, sleep, and movement practices. She had been an only child, carrying the full weight of caring for both of her aging parents. The timing was especially difficult, navigating a divorce while juggling a demanding job. Her high-stress levels over the years led to depression and coping habits like a few glasses of wine each night, microwaveable dinners, and falling asleep on the couch after late-night TV. She worked a sedentary job and had put on weight during menopause. She also admitted that the demands of life left little time for exercise or meaningful social connection.

Linda's symptoms weren't just about aging, they were about accumulation. Women often carry the weight of caregiving, career pressures, and emotional stress, all of which can take a toll on brain health over time. When we dug deeper, her lab results revealed low levels of estrogen, progesterone, and vitamin D3, along with elevated cortisol, blood sugar, lipids, liver function tests, and markers of inflammation. Her thyroid, B12, and folate levels were normal. Her brain MRI showed age-related atrophy signs and evidence of small vessel disease.

Linda's story is all too common. The perfect storm of genetic predisposition, chronic inflammation, hormonal shifts, metabolic imbalance, and lifestyle habits can set the stage for progressive cognitive issues over time. To properly address her brain health, we had to address the full picture of her physical, mental, and emotional well-being.

Linda's symptoms had physical causes, not just stress.

To truly understand why so many women like her experience brain fog, memory issues, and emotional shifts, we must look under the hood at what's happening in the female brain.

The Female Brain

Hormones: The Brain's Orchestra Conductor

Let us start with hormones. Our brain directly communicates with our ovaries, thyroid, and adrenal glands to make hormones. In return, those hormones circle back and signal to the brain when we have produced enough. This feedback loop is a two-way conversation: when our brain function shifts, it affects our hormones—and when our hormones change, it impacts our brain.

Many of us have felt this connection at different stages of life. During puberty, mood swings and trouble focusing often accompany hormonal shifts. In pregnancy, "pregnancy brain" can leave us feeling forgetful or foggy. And during menopause, it is as if the volume gets turned up on everything—hot flashes, sleep troubles, mood changes, and memory lapses can feel overwhelming. Our brain and body are navigating a storm, trying to find their footing as estrogen levels drop.

Speaking of estrogen, let us talk about this hormone's superhero role in the brain. Estrogen is like a shield, protecting our brain by enhancing memory, reducing inflammation, and even building new communication pathways between brain cells, a process known as neuroplasticity (the brain's ability to adapt and remodel itself over time).[37] It is also a powerful mood regulator, boosting feel-good chemicals like GABA (a calming neurotransmitter that helps reduce anxiety and promote relaxation),[38] dopamine, and endorphins, while fueling energy production and improving blood flow to the brain. Estrogen is the ultimate multitasker, keeping our brains sharp, stable, and resilient.

But after menopause, estrogen levels drop dramatically. Without this protective shield, the brain becomes more vulnerable to inflammation, energy dips, and cognitive decline. This is one of the reasons women are at higher risk for Alzheimer's and other forms of dementia post-menopause. It is like our brain has lost its best quarterback, and the game is not over yet.

From hormonal shifts to emotional stressors, another powerful player affecting the female brain is stress.

Stress: The Silent Brain Drain

Now, let us talk about stress, a constant companion for many of us. As women, we experience chronic stress differently than men, and it plays a major role in our brain health. When we are stressed, our adrenals release cortisol, the "stress hormone." In small doses, cortisol is helpful, it gives us the energy and focus to handle challenges. But when stress becomes chronic, and cortisol levels stay high for too long, it can wreak havoc on our brain, especially our memory center.

The hippocampus is our memory center. It stores and organizes memories and helps us learn new things. But when cortisol floods the system over time, it can shrink the hippocampus, making it harder to form new memories or recall old ones. Think of it like a computer running too many programs at once, it starts to slow down, glitch, or even crash.

For many of us, stress is a constant part of life. We juggle careers, caregiving, relationships, and societal pressures, often putting our own needs last. This kind of ongoing stress weighs us down, and over time, it takes a toll on our brain health. Women are more prone to anxiety and depression, which are closely linked to high cortisol levels. The way we process stress, often internalizing it or ruminating on it, can make us more vulnerable to its long-term impacts.

Stress can wear us down over time, but it is not the only invisible threat to our cognitive health. Let us look at another major culprit that is often overlooked: inflammation.

Inflammation: The Hidden Fire in Your Brain

Another factor that can harm our brain health is inflammation. Think of inflammation like a fire in your body. In small, controlled amounts, inflammation is helpful. It is how your body heals itself like when you get a cut or a bruise. But when inflammation becomes chronic and out of control, it is like a wildfire that just keeps spreading, damaging everything in its path.

In the brain, chronic inflammation can harm neurons, disrupt communication between brain cells, and even lead to the buildup of harmful proteins like amyloid plaques, which are linked to Alzheimer's disease. Over time, this can cause memory loss, brain fog, and other cognitive issues.

What causes brain inflammation? For starters, autoimmune conditions, which are much more common in women, can trigger chronic inflammation. Conditions like lupus, rheumatoid arthritis, Hashimoto's thyroiditis, and multiple sclerosis (MS) can cause inflammation in the brain. Other factors include diabetes, high blood pressure, and high cholesterol, issues that many women face, especially after menopause.

Everyday habits can also fuel brain inflammation. Eating ultra-processed foods, skimping on sleep, or chronic stress can trigger body-wide inflammation, including in the brain. Even alcohol consumption and smoking can harm your brain, damaging blood vessels and reducing blood flow. We now know even one alcoholic drink can put our brains at risk.

And let us not forget environmental factors. Exposure to chemicals, toxins, chronic infections, or even mold can slowly chip away at your brain health, causing inflammation and oxidative stress over time.

This brings us to a powerful, often underestimated ally in brain health: your body's gut-brain connection. Let us look at how your brain relies on it to function at its best.

The Brain-Gut Connection: Your Second Brain

Now, let us explore one of the most exciting areas of health science: the brain-gut connection. Did you know your gut is often called your "second brain"? It is home to the enteric nervous system, a complex network of neurons that communicate directly with your brain via the Vagus nerve. This two-way communication system is why you feel "butterflies" when you are nervous or why stress can upset your stomach.

But the gut-brain connection goes even deeper, thanks to the microbiome, the trillions of bacteria, viruses, and fungi living in your gut. These microbes play a crucial role in your brain health. They produce neurotransmitters like serotonin (often called the "happy hormone"), which regulates mood, sleep, and appetite. About 90% of serotonin and 50% of dopamine is made in the gut![39]

When your microbiome is out of balance, a condition called dysbiosis, it can lead to inflammation, mood disorders, and even cognitive decline. Research shows that an unhealthy gut microbiome is linked to conditions like anxiety, depression, and Alzheimer's disease.

So, how can you support your gut-brain axis? Start by eating a diet rich in fiber, fermented foods, and prebiotics (which feed your good bacteria). Avoid processed foods, excess sugar, and artificial sweeteners, which can harm your microbiome. And do not forget about oral health, your mouth is the gateway to your gut, and poor oral hygiene can lead to an imbalance in your microbiome. Brushing, flossing, and regular dental check-ups are essential for maintaining a healthy gut and brain.

As we have seen, the health of our gut, immune system, hormones, and daily habits all feed into a bigger picture. But knowledge is only powerful when it leads to action. So, what does it look like to take proactive steps toward protecting our brain health, especially as women? Let us revisit Linda's journey to see what is possible.

The Power of Prevention

Linda's journey started with her desire to improve her brain health. Together, we crafted a plan to tackle her metabolic issues, blood sugar, cholesterol, and hormones through a combination of medications, supplements, and lifestyle changes. She started small, with manageable steps like adding a daily walk, cutting back on processed foods, and practicing mindfulness to manage stress. Over time, we set goals for better sleep, stronger social connections, stress-relief activities, resistance training, and the MIND diet (which we explore next), all of which helped improve her blood sugar, weight, and inflammatory markers.

Gradually, Linda noticed improvements in her memory, focus, and overall well-being. Her story is a powerful reminder that while we cannot change our genetics, we can take meaningful steps to protect our brain health and reduce the risk of cognitive decline. By understanding the unique factors that impact women's brain health, we can make informed choices that build cognitive resilience and support a vibrant, healthy mind for years to come.

Now that you have seen how lifestyle changes helped Linda reclaim her cognitive health, let us talk about how you can take proactive steps too. The truth is many of the most powerful tools for protecting your brain are already within your reach.

What You Can Do: Protecting Your Brain Health

The good news is that much of our brain health is in our hands. By making simple, brain-healthy lifestyle changes, we can lower our risk of cognitive decline and strengthen our mental resilience for the years ahead. Let us break it down into seven key areas: nutrition, exercise, sleep, stress management, social connections, hormone therapy, and environmental factors.

1. Nourish Your Brain: The MIND Diet

Have you heard of the MIND diet? Research shows that following this diet can slash your risk of Alzheimer's by a jaw-dropping 53%.[40] That is not just impressive, it is a total game-changer for your brain health. No drug ever has dropped the risk of Alzheimer's by 53%.

MIND stands for *Mediterranean-DASH Intervention for Neurodegenerative Delay*, and it combines the best of the Mediterranean and DASH diets. Studies like the groundbreaking FINGER trial (*Finnish Geriatric Intervention Study to Prevent Cognitive Impairment and Disability*) have shown just how powerful this diet can be for protecting your brain.[41]

So, what did the FINGER study find? Researchers followed 1,260 older adults at risk of cognitive decline.[42] Those who ate a brain-healthy diet, exercised regularly, engaged in cognitive training, and managed vascular risk factors (like blood pressure and cholesterol) saw significant improvements in memory and thinking skills. The takeaway? Think about what you eat, how you move, and how you care for your body all working together to keep your brain sharp and resilient.

1. What to Eat on the MIND Diet

The MIND Diet is all about nourishing your mind, and these are the stars of the show:

- **Leafy Greens** (Spinach, Kale, Swiss Chard, etc.)
  Think of these as your brain's best friends. Aim for at least six servings a week. They are loaded with brain-boosting nutrients like folate, vitamin K, and antioxidants. Toss them into salads, blend them into smoothies, or sauté them with a little olive oil and garlic for a quick, delicious side.

- **Berries** (Blueberries, Strawberries, Raspberries, etc.)
Who does not love berries? Try to enjoy two or more servings a week. These little gems are packed with flavonoids, which help protect your brain cells and even improve memory. Add them to your yogurt, sprinkle them on oatmeal, or just snack on them as they are.
- **Nuts** (Almonds, Walnuts, Pistachios, etc.)
A small handful (about an ounce) of nuts a day is all you need. They are a great source of healthy fats, vitamin E, and antioxidants, all of which are great for your brain. Walnuts are especially powerful due to their high omega-3 fatty content.
- **Whole Grains** (Quinoa, Oats, Brown Rice, Whole Wheat, etc.)
Make whole grains a daily staple and aim for at least three servings a day. They are rich in fiber, B vitamins, and antioxidants, which help reduce inflammation and keep your brain functioning at its best. Swap out refined grains (like white bread) for whole-grain options whenever you can.
- **Fatty Fish (Salmon, Mackerel, Sardines, Trout, etc.)**
Aim for at least one serving per week. These are loaded with omega-3 fatty acids (DHA and EPA), which are essential for brain health and reducing inflammation. Grill, bake or steam your fish for a healthy and satisfying meal.
- **Low-fat dairy (Yogurt, Milk, Cheese, etc.)**
Include one to two servings of low-fat dairy daily. It is a great source of calcium and vitamin D, which are important for overall health. Stick to plain, unsweetened yogurt or low-fat milk.
- **Olive Oil**
Make olive oil your go-to cooking oil. It is rich in monounsaturated fats and polyphenols, which protect brain cells and reduce inflammation. Drizzle it over salads or use it for light sautéing, it is a simple way to boost your brain health.

- **Beans and legumes**
  Aim for at least four servings a week. They are a source of plant-based protein and nutrients that support metabolic and brain health.
- **Poultry** (Chicken, Turkey)
  The MIND Diet recommends two or more servings per week as a healthy protein source that may benefit cognitive function.

2. What to Limit or Avoid on the MIND Diet

Now, let us talk about the foods that do not do your brain any favors. For some of these foods, moderation is key:

- **Red Meat:** Try to limit it to no more than three servings a week. High intake has been linked to inflammation and cognitive decline.
- **Butter and Spreads:** Use these sparingly, less than a tablespoon a day. Olive oil is a much better choice.
- **Full-Fat Cheese:** Keep it to less than one serving a week.
- **Ultra-Processed Foods and Fried Foods:** Cut out these foods high in unhealthy fats and additives that can harm your brain.
- **Refined Flour and Sugar**: Cut out white bread, pastries, and sweets, these can spike your blood sugar and increase inflammation.
- **Alcohol**: Too much alcohol can be harmful to your brain. Some studies show that even one drink a week can have negative effects on the brain.

Why It Works:

The MIND diet focuses on foods that reduce inflammation, protect brain cells, and improve blood flow to the brain. By combining the best of the Mediterranean and DASH diets, it is designed to support long-term cognitive health and reduce the risk of Alzheimer's and dementia.

Let us keep building on that momentum by looking at another powerful brain booster: movement. What you do with your body can have just as much impact as what you put on your plate.

2. Move Your Body: Exercise and Brain Health

Did you know that moving your body can protect your brain? A study in *Neurology* found that older adults who did regular aerobic exercise had a 50% lower risk of dementia compared to those who were less active.[43] How does this work? It is all about the amazing connection between your muscles and brain. When you move, your muscles release special chemicals (myokines), called BDNF, that travel to your brain. These chemicals, like fertilizer, help grow new brain cells, reduce inflammation, and keep your mind sharp. When you exercise regularly, it increases the size of the hippocampus, the part of your brain responsible for memory. Plus, exercise reduces inflammation, which is a big contributor to brain diseases.

So, what kind of exercise should you do to protect your brain? Here is a science-backed plan to get started:

1. Aerobic Exercise

Aim for 150 minutes of moderate-intensity exercise per week, which is about 30 minutes, 5 days a week. Activities like brisk walking, swimming, cycling, or even dancing are all fantastic choices.

2. Strength Training

Incorporate resistance exercises 2-3 times a week. Strength training is not just about building muscle, it also supports brain health by improving insulin sensitivity and reducing inflammation.

3. Mind-Body Exercises

Try yoga or tai chi for a perfect blend of movement and mindfulness. These practices not only reduce stress and improve balance but also boost brain health. A 2019 study in *The Journal of Alzheimer's Disease* found that tai chi improved cognitive function and even increased brain volume in older adults.[44]

4. Daily Walking

Do not underestimate the power of a simple daily walk. Even 20-30 minutes a day can do wonders for your mood, memory, and cognitive function. A study from the University of Pittsburgh found that walking 6-9 miles per week reduced brain shrinkage and helped preserve memory in older adults.[45]

The key is to start small and build consistency. Begin with a 10-minute walk or a short yoga session and gradually increase your activity level. Most importantly, find activities you enjoy, because sticking with them long-term is one of the most powerful ways to protect your cognitive health and reduce your risk of dementia.

Just like movement is fuel for your brain, sleep is the foundation that keeps everything functioning smoothly. Let us take a look at why rest is one of the most powerful tools you have for brain longevity.

3. Prioritize Sleep: The Foundation of Brain Health

Sleep is not just something you do when you have time, it is non-negotiable for your brain health. Think of it as your brain's nightly reset button. Women who sleep less than six hours nightly have three times higher Alzheimer's risk, because during deep sleep, your brain flushes out toxic proteins like amyloid-beta.[46] Skip just 90 minutes of sleep, and these plaques surge 30%, silently erasing your memories.[47] Meanwhile, late-night scrolling? It is the equivalent of drinking three shots of espresso before bed, slashing deep sleep by 58%. So, if you are ignoring sleep, it is time to rethink your habits.[48]

Here are six practical tips to help you sleep better and protect your brain:

1. Stick to a Schedule

Your brain loves routine. Try to go to bed and wake up at the same time every day, even on weekends. Get 15 minutes of morning sunlight to help regulate your circadian rhythm.

2. Create a Sleep-Friendly Space

Turn your bedroom into a sleep sanctuary. Keep it cool, dark, and quiet. If your mattress or pillows are past their prime, consider investing in new ones.

3. Limit Screens Before Bed

That blue light from your phone, tablet, or TV? It is a melatonin killer. Try to power down your devices 1-2 hours before bedtime.

4. Wind Down with a Routine

Create a calming pre-sleep ritual. Read a book, take a warm bath, or do some gentle yoga. These activities signal to your brain that it is time to relax and unwind.

5. Avoid Stimulants

Caffeine and alcohol might seem like your friends, but they can wreak havoc on your sleep, especially if you consume them in the afternoon or evening. Try to cut back and see how it impacts your rest.

6. Supplements

If you are still struggling with sleep, consider some evidence-based supplements that might help. Options to explore include magnesium glycinate, melatonin, L-theanine, GABA, and tart cherry juice. Always consult your healthcare provider to ensure they are safe and right for you!

Why It Matters

Poor sleep is not just about feeling groggy, it is linked to cognitive decline and Alzheimer's. Address any concerns of sleep apnea with your doctor and get tested. By prioritizing sleep, you protect your brain and boost your memory, focus, and overall brain health. Combine good sleep hygiene with evidence-based tools, and you will give your brain the rest it needs to thrive.

You have learned how sleep resets and recharges your brain, but what happens when stress keeps your mind in overdrive? Let us talk about the next pillar of brain health: learning how to manage stress before it hijacks your memory and mental clarity.

4. Manage Stress: Meditation and Brain Health

Let us talk about stress. It is not just a mental burden; it is a major threat to your brain health. As we have discussed, when you are stressed, your body releases cortisol, a hormone that, over time, can damage your memory, emotional regulation, and cognitive function. Prolonged stress does not just make you feel frazzled; it can shrink your hippocampus (the part of your brain critical for memory), impair your prefrontal cortex (responsible for decision-making), and disrupt communication between brain cells. All of this can accelerate cognitive decline.

The good news? You can fight back with some powerful, science-backed tools. Here's how to manage stress and protect your brain:

1. Mindfulness Meditation

Meditation is for anyone who wants to protect their brain. Maybe you have thought of starting a meditation practice but struggle with knowing where to start. A simple practice can be walking meditation, where you pay attention to your surroundings with all your senses in nature. Another way is to pay attention to all four parts of your breath cycle: when you breathe in, the pause, when you breathe out, and then the pause. Mindfulness meditation reduces anxiety and depression, both of which can worsen cognitive decline. Regular meditation can help you form new neural connections.

A notable study conducted by Harvard researchers explored the effects of Kirtan Kriya, a form of meditation rooted in Kundalini yoga, on Alzheimer's patients.[49] The study found that practicing Kirtan Kriya for just 12 minutes a day over eight weeks led to significant improvements in memory, cognitive function, and overall brain health. Participants also showed increased blood flow to areas of the brain associated with memory and emotional regulation. This research highlights the profound impact that even short, consistent meditation practices can have on brain health, particularly for those at risk of or experiencing cognitive decline.

2. Yoga

Yoga lowers cortisol levels and increases gray matter, which improves cognition and emotional regulation. Plus, the breathwork involved in yoga activates your parasympathetic nervous system, helping you feel calm and centered.

3. Forest Bathing (Shinrin-Yoku)

Yes, "forest bathing" is amazing for your brain. Spending time in nature reduces cortisol, lowers blood pressure, and improves your mood. A 2019 study in Environmental Health and Preventive Medicine found that forest bathing even boosts immune function and reduces stress hormones.[50] Even just 20-30 minutes in a green space can significantly lower your cortisol levels. So, take a walk in the park or sit under a tree, your brain will thank you.

4. Deep Breathing

Sometimes, the simplest tools are the most effective. Deep breathing techniques, like diaphragmatic breathing or the 4-7-8 method (inhale for 4, hold for 7, exhale for 8), activate your body's relaxation response. This lowers cortisol levels and improves mental clarity. It is like hitting a reset button for your brain.

By managing stress with these evidence-based tools, you are not just protecting your brain, you are enhancing cognitive function and supporting long-term brain health.

Let us look at the next key area of brain protection, one that is surprisingly powerful: your social life.

5. Stay Socially Connected: The Link Between Isolation and Dementia

Did you know that staying socially connected is not just good for your mood, it is essential for your brain health? Social isolation is a significant risk factor for cognitive decline and dementia, and research shows just how damaging loneliness can be. Studies have found that loneliness increases stress, inflammation, and the risk of depression, all of which can speed up cognitive decline.

For example, a study published in *The Journal of Aging and Health* found that isolated individuals had a 40% higher risk of developing dementia compared to those with strong social connections.[51] And social isolation can even shrink the brain, particularly the hippocampus, which is crucial for memory and learning.

One major contributor to social isolation? Hearing loss. When people struggle to hear, they often withdraw from conversations or avoid social situations altogether. This withdrawal can accelerate cognitive decline and an increased risk of dementia.

So, what can you do to protect your brain? Here are some practical steps:

1. Get Regular Hearing Check-Ups

If you have noticed any changes in your hearing, do not wait, get it checked. Using hearing aids, if needed, can make a world of difference in staying connected and engaged.

2. Stay Socially Active

Staying engaged in social activities is critical for your mental well-being. Join clubs, volunteer, or take classes where you can meet new people.

3. Nurture Relationships

Make time for the people who matter most. Schedule regular calls or visits with friends and family. Even small, consistent efforts to stay connected can have a big impact.

4. Participate in Group Activities

Whether it is a book club, an exercise class, or a community event, group activities keep you mentally sharp while helping you build meaningful connections.

Staying socially engaged is about having fun and it is a vital part of your brain health puzzle.

6. Clean Up Your Environment: The Impact of Toxins on Brain Health

Environmental toxins can have a significant impact on brain health, especially for women. Studies show that exposure to chemicals found in everyday products, like pesticides, heavy metals, skincare, beauty products, makeup, perfumes, and cookware, can increase the risk of cognitive decline and other health issues. These substances can interfere with hormone balance and brain function, posing a particular risk to women to our unique hormonal biology.

The good news? You can start reducing your exposure today with a few intentional shifts. Here are some simple yet powerful ways to protect your brain by creating a cleaner, safer environment:

1. Choose Organic Produce

Opt for organic fruits and vegetables whenever possible to minimize pesticide exposure. Pesticides have been linked to neurotoxicity and cognitive decline. Not sure where to start? Check out the *Dirty Dozen* list at EWG.org to find the twelve most heavily pesticide-loaded produce on the market and buy these organic when possible.

2. Filter Your Water

Use a high-quality water filter to reduce your exposure to heavy metals like lead and mercury, which can negatively impact brain health.

3. Switch to Clean Beauty Products

When it comes to skincare and makeup, choose products labeled "paraben-free" and "phthalate-free." Use apps like *Yuka* (yuka.io) and *Think Dirty* (thinkdirtyapp.com) to find safer, non-toxic brands and products.

4. Avoid Synthetic Fragrances

Many perfumes and scented products contain hormone-disrupting chemicals. Opt for natural or non-toxic fragrances.

5. Upgrade Your Cookware

Avoid non-stick pans that release harmful chemicals (like PFAS) when heated. Instead, choose safer alternatives like stainless steel, cast iron, or ceramic cookware.

6. Support Your Body's Natural Detoxification

You do not need a fancy detox to stay healthy. Focus on a clean diet rich in antioxidants, drink plenty of water, regulate your bowels, and exercise regularly to help your body naturally eliminate toxins.

By making these small but impactful changes, you can significantly reduce your exposure to environmental toxins, protect your brain health, and support your overall well-being, inside and out.

Suggested Supplements for Brain Health

Supporting your brain health goes beyond diet and exercise, certain evidence-based supplements have shown promise in supporting cognitive function, protecting against age-related decline, and reducing the risk of neurodegenerative diseases like Alzheimer's. However, these supplements should not replace a healthy lifestyle, but they can serve as powerful allies in your wellness toolkit. As always, consult your healthcare provider before starting any new supplement, especially if you have any underlying conditions or take medications. See Appendix B for a list of these recommended supplements for brain health.

Final Thoughts

Women's brain health is multifaced, but it does not have to feel overwhelming. The more you understand the critical roles of hormones, inflammation, stress, sleep, and lifestyle, the more empowered you can become to care for your mind in a holistic and proactive way.

Your brain is your most precious asset. It deserves the same attention and care you give to your heart, your hormones, and the rest of your body. Through the strategies shared in this chapter, whether it is optimizing your diet, getting regular exercise, improving sleep, managing stress, or exploring hormone therapy, you now have a toolbox to help you thrive, not just survive.

Let us stop dismissing memory lapses and brain fog as "just part of getting older." Instead, I want you to feel empowered to take control of your brain health. You can strengthen and support your brain at every stage of life.

A healthy brain is the foundation for a vibrant, fulfilling life, and it is never too early or too late to start prioritizing it.

Questions To Discuss With Your Doctor:

These questions are designed to help you have a more informed, collaborative conversation with your healthcare provider, so you can get to the root of what is going on and build a plan that supports your mental, emotional, and physical well-being.

1. Can I get lab work to assess my brain health?

Consider: CBC, CMP, thyroid panel, vitamin D3, homocysteine, fasting insulin, glucose, lipids, ApoE genotype, hs-CRP, IL-6, HbA1c, hormone panel, F2-isoprostanes, 8-OHdG, TNF-alpha, IL-1beta, heavy metals, B12, folate, MTHFR, and celiac/gluten sensitivity testing.

2. Would imaging like an MRI, PET, or SPECT scan be helpful to evaluate my brain health?

These tests can provide insights into brain structure, function, and potential areas of concern.

> **3. Is there a specialist we can consult for neurocognitive testing?**

Neurocognitive assessments can help identify early signs of cognitive decline or memory issues.

> **4. Are there any vitamins or supplements that could support my brain health?**

Consider: Methylated B vitamins, vitamin D3, omega-3 fatty acids, curcumin, L-carnitine, CoQ10, alpha-lipoic acid (ALA), and magnesium.

> **5. Can we test for nutrient deficiencies that might be impacting my brain function?**

Consider: Vitamin D, B vitamins, magnesium, zinc, and omega-3 fatty acids.

> **6. Would it be helpful to assess my gut health, given its connection to brain health?**

Consider: Stool testing for dysbiosis, leaky gut markers, and microbiome diversity.

> **7. Can we evaluate my stress and adrenal health, as chronic stress can impact cognitive function?**

Consider: Cortisol testing through saliva to assess adrenal function and stress impact.

8. Are there lifestyle changes we can focus on to support my brain health?

Discuss: Stress management techniques, sleep optimization, exercise, and dietary changes like the MIND diet.

9. Can we partner together to create a preventative health plan for my brain health?

Work with your doctor to develop a personalized plan that addresses your unique needs and goals.

For a complete companion resource, including all "Questions to Discuss with Your Doctor," Supplement Lists, and Guides, scan the QR code.

Chapter 5

Mental Health

"It's not stress that kills us, it is our reaction to it."

—**Hans Selye**

Stress. That is a word that has defined so much of my life. Through medical school and residency, I wore it like a badge of honor, working long hours, sleepless nights, meals scarfed down between patients, and a constant pressure to prove myself. As women, we are taught to push harder, to be stronger, to outwork and outlast, especially in spaces where we are surrounded by men. As an Internal Medicine-Pediatrics resident, I was no exception. Completing two residences at the same time, I felt the weight of needing to show up bigger, smarter, and more resilient than ever, just to be seen as equal.

Even after residency, I thought the finish line was in sight. I told myself, *just get through this, and life will slow down*. But the truth is, the hamster wheel never stops. It just changes shape. My first job as a full-fledged doctor brought a new kind of pressure: more responsibility, more decisions, more lives depending on me. And then came the leap of starting my own practice. It was supposed to be my dream, my chance to build something meaningful. But with it came a mountain of paperwork, sleepless nights worrying about payroll, and the constant juggle of managing a team while still being present for my patients.

And then there was home. I would wake up running from the moment my feet hit the floor. Breakfasts to make, lunches to pack, kids to get to school, and a never-ending to-do list that seemed to grow faster than I could check things off. I was a wife, a mother, a daughter, and a friend, roles I cherished, but roles that demanded so much of me. Everyone needed something, and I wanted to give it to them. But while tending to everyone else's needs, I lost sight of my own. The impact of all of this took a serious toll on my health, but I was too busy to see the connection... until I did.

This is not just my story; it is the story of countless women. Doctors, teachers, lawyers, mothers, corporate CEOs, the list goes on, we carry the invisible burden of stress every single day. We are expected to juggle it all, to keep going no matter the cost. And while we may have a remarkable capacity to endure, the toll it takes on us is profound. Stress does not just live in our minds; it seeps into our bodies. It disrupts our hormones, weakens our immune systems, and wreaks havoc on our digestive and reproductive health.

Why Women Feel Stuck

To understand the full impact of stress, we must explore the deeper patterns that keep women in survival mode.

Chronic stress can cause disease, and disease can cause stress. It is a vicious cycle, and for women, it is even harder to break because too often, we are not taken seriously when we seek help.

I have seen this over and over in my practice. Women come to me exhausted, in pain, or just feeling "off," only to be told by other doctors, "It's just stress." Yes, stress can make us sick, but being sick can also make us stressed. And when doctors dismiss our symptoms as "all in our heads," it does not just delay treatment, it erodes trust and leaves us feeling invisible.

A Patient Story: Kelly's Journey – When Pain and Trauma Collide

Let me tell you about Kelly. She is a 53-year-old woman whose life changed in an instant. One moment, she was driving on the interstate; the next, a large truck rear-ended her at 65 mph. The impact left her with devastating injuries to her neck and back. But the aftermath? That was worse. Chronic pain. Debilitating headaches. Pelvic floor dysfunction. And the haunting grip of post-traumatic stress that followed her everywhere.

At first, Kelly tried to tough it out. She didn't want to be a burden, so she downplayed her pain. She relied on ibuprofen and home stretches, hoping it would all just go away. But it didn't. The pain got worse, and so did her anxiety. She lived in constant fear of having stool incontinence in public. She avoided social gatherings or outings, worried she wouldn't be able to walk back to her car because of the pain. Even the thought of getting into a car sent her into a panic.

When Kelly finally sought help, she was met with dismissal. Doctors minimized her suffering, chalking her symptoms up to anxiety. They brushed off her pelvic pain and rectal pressure as if they didn't matter. No one was truly listening.

It was not until her spine MRI returned that the truth became undeniable. The scans showed significant injuries that could not be ignored. Surgeons recommended aggressive spinal surgeries, but the thought of going under the knife filled Kelly with fear. She was terrified of paralysis, disability, and even death. Yet, the daily toll of her pain was unbearable. It stole her sleep, left her with heart palpitations, shattered her concentration, led to weight gain, and plunged her into a deep depression. She felt stuck, caught between the rock of her pain and the hard place of her fear.

This is where our journey together began. Kelly was searching for another way, a gentler, less invasive path to heal her body and reclaim her life. She was determined to leave no stone unturned, exploring every possibility to find relief from her physical pain. But she also knew the trauma, fear, anxiety, the emotional scars she carried also needed healing. For Kelly, true healing meant addressing the whole picture, not just the pieces.

Kelly's story is a powerful reminder of how deeply our mental health is tied to our physical bodies, especially for women. We carry so much, the weight of our pain, the stress of caring for others, and the guilt of feeling like we are never enough. Unlike men, we tend to internalize stress more deeply, and it can worsen physical symptoms like headaches, digestive issues, and chronic pain.

But here's the problem: when we share our anxiety with doctors, it is often used to explain away our symptoms instead of recognizing it as a biological reaction to our illness. This is why healing our minds is just as important as healing our bodies. For women, the two are intertwined. When we address anxiety, depression, and trauma, we create space for our bodies to follow.

Kelly's journey is far from over, but she has already made incredible strides. By confronting her PTSD (post-traumatic stress disorder) and exploring integrative approaches to her pain, she started to reclaim her life. Her story is a testament to the power of addressing the whole person— body, mind, and spirit.

As women, we deserve to be heard, believed, and treated as more than just a collection of symptoms. We deserve care that recognizes the deep connection between our physical and emotional health.

Now, let us look at how this connection plays out inside the body. In the next section, we will explore the biology of stress and how it shows up in real, physical ways, and why a personalized approach is essential to healing.

Our Stress Response: Fight, Flight, Freeze

Kelly's story is a powerful reminder of how illness and stress can collide, creating a cycle that feels impossible to break. But to truly understand what's happening in our bodies, and why stress impacts women so deeply, we need to start with the basics. Let us break it down.

Imagine you are walking in the woods at night, and suddenly, you hear a rustle in the bushes. Your heart races, your breath quickens, your muscles tense, and your stomach drops. You are frozen, convinced it is a bear. This is your body's fight, flight, or freeze response kicking in. It is like an internal alarm system designed to keep you alive. Your brain screams, *Danger!* and floods your body with stress hormones like cortisol and adrenaline. Blood rushes to your heart, lungs, and muscles, preparing you to fight or run, while your digestion, immune system, and even your reproductive system take a backseat. Survival comes first.

But what happens when we face stress every day, whether it is a sudden crisis or a slow-building burden? Our bodies react in ways that are hardwired for survival. But when the "danger" does not go away, when the stress becomes chronic—day after day, week after week, year after year—our systems stay on high alert.

Most of us are not running from bears. Instead, we are dealing with a virtual bear, the one that follows us from the moment we wake up to the moment we (try to) sleep. It is the stress of deadlines, traffic, finances, relationships, and the endless to-do lists that keep us in a constant state of hyper-alertness. This virtual bear keeps our bodies stuck in fight or flight mode, activating the sympathetic nervous system, leaving no room for the other side of our nervous system, the rest and digest mode, to do its job.

This calmer side, the parasympathetic nervous system, is run by the Vagus nerve, a superhighway in your body that helps you relax, digest food, fight off infections, and even repair your cells. It is like the *off switch* for stress. But when we are constantly stressed, the Vagus nerve shuts down, and our bodies cannot recover. Over time, this leads to mood swings, digestive issues, weight gain, frequent colds, and so much more.

The good news? You are not stuck here. There are practical ways to shift your nervous system out of stress mode and back into a state of healing and calm. Up next, we will talk about how stress shows up in the body and how you can begin to shift the balance in your favor.

Stress and Inflammation

And here is where it gets even more complicated for us as women: stress does not just keep us on edge, it fuels inflammation in our bodies. When we are stressed, cortisol is supposed to help regulate inflammation, but when stress becomes chronic, those cortisol levels can go haywire. Instead of calming inflammation, cortisol can make it worse. This combination of stress and inflammation creates a vicious cycle that hits women harder than men.

Why? Stress can amplify inflammatory responses, making us more susceptible to conditions like autoimmune diseases, which include lupus, rheumatoid arthritis, or Hashimoto's thyroiditis. Chronic stress can also disrupt our gut health, leading to issues like irritable bowel syndrome (IBS) or leaky gut, which further fuels inflammation. And because our hormonal systems are especially sensitive, stress impacts our reproductive health too, disrupting ovulation, worsening PMS, and even contributing to conditions like PCOS and endometriosis, which are deeply tied to inflammation.

Over time, this stress-inflammation combo can lead to systemic inflammation, a silent fire that spreads throughout the body. It is linked to high blood pressure, heart disease, diabetes, and even mental health issues like depression and anxiety. For women, this is especially dangerous because we are already at higher risk for autoimmune diseases, hormonal imbalances, and conditions like fibromyalgia, all of which are rooted in inflammation.

The more we understand how stress affects our bodies, the better we can break the cycle. But stress does not just cause inflammation, it can also trigger weight gain, making it harder to lose stubborn pounds. Let us look at why this happens and how to reclaim control.

Stress and Weight Gain

We have all been there. We have all experienced the frustration of trying to lose weight, only to hit a wall no matter how hard we try. We start a weight loss journey, fully committed—counting every calorie, sweating through intense workouts, and saying no to the foods we love—only to watch the scale barely budge. Meanwhile, the men in our lives seem to shed pounds effortlessly, as if by magic. It's frustrating, isn't it? But what no one tells you is that it is not just willpower or effort. Our bodies are wired differently, especially when it comes to stress and weight.

Here's what no one tells us: when we push ourselves too hard through intense workouts, restrictive diets, or long, exhausting workdays, we are working against our biology. These habits can backfire because our bodies are designed to store fat during stressful times. It is a survival mechanism, deeply rooted in our biology. When we are stressed, whether it is emotional turmoil, physical strain, from over-exercising, or fasting, our bodies release cortisol. And for women, high cortisol does not just leave us feeling anxious or on edge; it signals our bodies to hold onto fat, especially around the abdomen. Evolutionarily, this was meant to protect us (and potential pregnancies) during tough times.

And it gets even more interesting. Our X chromosome influences how we store fat, manage insulin, and regulate metabolism. This makes us more prone to insulin resistance and visceral fat retention when cortisol is high. So, when we are stressed or going through hormonal changes like PMS, perimenopause, or postpartum, our bodies are more likely to cling to fat, no matter how hard we are trying to lose it. It is not just about willpower; it is about how our bodies are wired to respond to stress.

This is why the traditional "eat less, move more" approach often fails us. When we push ourselves with punishing workouts, restrictive diets, or long hours without rest, we are actually spiking our cortisol levels and essentially telling our bodies to hold onto fat. It is a vicious cycle, and it is not your fault. You have just been given the wrong playbook.

So, what's the solution? It is time to stop fighting against our bodies and start working with them. Instead of intense cardio or calorie counting, we can focus on strength training, which builds muscle and supports metabolism without spiking cortisol. Instead of fasting or skipping meals, we can prioritize nourishing, balanced meals that keep our blood sugar stable. Instead of pushing through exhaustion, we can give ourselves permission to rest, say "no" to things that drain us, and practice stress management techniques like deep breathing, yoga, or even just taking a walk in nature.

Our bodies are incredible, resilient, and uniquely ours. They are not designed to be punished; they are designed to be nurtured. By understanding how stress and hormones impact us, we can create a healthier, more sustainable path to well-being. It is not about perfection or pushing harder; it is about giving ourselves grace and working with our biology, not against it.

Next, let us explore how stress affects our digestion, because what happens in our gut is often the first sign that our body is feeling overwhelmed.

Stress and Digestion

Every time I travel, without fail, my digestion goes haywire. It takes days, sometimes even a week, to get back on track. The same thing happens when I am juggling a big project at work or navigating a particularly hectic week. Sound familiar? It is like your gut has a mind of its own, and it knows when life gets overwhelming. For some of us, stress sends our bowels into overdrive, leading to diarrhea. For others, it is the opposite, everything just shuts down, leaving us bloated, uncomfortable, and, well, constipated.

This frustrating connection between stress and digestion comes down to what's often called our "second brain", the enteric nervous system. Your gut has its own nervous system, and its star player is the Vagus nerve. This powerful nerve is like the conductor of your digestive orchestra, regulating everything from the saliva in your mouth to the acid in your stomach, the bile released by your liver and gallbladder, the digestive enzymes from your pancreas, and even the health of the trillions of bacteria in your colon (your microbiome). But when stress hits, the Vagus nerve essentially goes offline. It is like the conductor has left the building and the whole orchestra falls out of sync.

And for us women, this stress-gut connection tends to hit harder. We are more likely to experience gas, bloating, abdominal pain, indigestion, constipation, or diarrhea when life gets overwhelming. In fact, 60-70% of all IBS (Irritable Bowel Syndrome) diagnoses are in women.[52] But here's the thing: IBS is often a catch-all term, a label we reach for when we do not fully understand what is causing the problem or how to fix it. The truth is, many of our digestive issues are rooted in stress and how it impacts our bodies differently than men's.

As women, understanding how stress affects our digestion is the first step to feeling better. When we recognize how deeply our emotional and physiological responses disrupt gut function, we can begin to address the true root of the problem. Managing stress and supporting gut health go hand in hand, and doing so creates a more stable, vibrant, and balanced life.

Managing stress and supporting gut health go hand in hand, but this connection extends far beyond digestion alone. The same Vagus nerve that regulates your gut also controls your hormonal balance, reproductive health, and stress response system.

Next, let us explore how chronic stress disrupts this delicate hormonal orchestra, and what that means for your body's natural rhythms.

Stress and Hormones

Imagine a rabbit in the wild, darting through the trees as a pack of wolves closes in. She is not thinking about having babies, she is focused on survival. Her body knows reproduction is a luxury for calmer times. Reproduction is controlled by the Vagus nerve, which also manages our digestion, emotions, and hormones. When we are stressed, this nerve puts non-essential functions, like reproduction, on pause until we feel safe again.

Now, as modern women, we are not running from literal wolves, but our bodies react the same way to stress. Whether it is juggling kids, working, or just trying to breathe, our bodies see it all as dangerous. When we are stuck in this stressed-out mode, our Vagus nerve shuts down systems like fertility and hormonal balance.

Stress triggers cortisol, which messes with our reproductive hormones, especially estrogen and progesterone needed for ovulation and a healthy menstrual cycle. Chronic stress can stop ovulation, cause irregular periods, or even make them disappear. For women with PCOS, stress can worsen insulin resistance, causing weight gain, acne, and unwanted hair. For those with endometriosis, stress increases inflammation, making pain worse. And for anyone with PMS or PMDD, stress can turn a tough week into an emotional nightmare.

But the hormonal disruption does not end there. Stress can also mess with your thyroid. High cortisol can slow thyroid function, leaving you tired, sluggish, and struggling with weight gain. This is because cortisol messes with how your body uses thyroid hormones, putting your metabolism on hold.

The bottom line? Stress and hormones are deeply connected. When we understand how stress affects our cycles, worsens conditions like PCOS or endometriosis, and disrupts thyroid function, we can start to take back control. By managing stress and supporting our hormones, we can feel more balanced, energized, and healthy.

But this stress response does not stop there, it cascades through every system in your body, including one of your most vital defenses: your immune system.

Just as stress throws off hormonal balance, it also weakens our immunity, leaving us vulnerable when we need protection most. Let us examine why this happens.

Stress and Immunity

Have you ever noticed that during particularly stressful times, you seem to catch every cold, flu, or infection that comes your way? That is not a coincidence. When stress takes over, our bodies prioritize survival over everything else, including our immune system. Just like we have seen with digestion, hormones, and inflammation, stress has a profound impact on how well our bodies can fight off illness.

When we perceive a threat, whether it is a looming deadline, a family crisis, or even just the daily grind, our brain triggers the release of stress hormones like cortisol. In small doses, cortisol can help regulate inflammation and support immune function. But when stress becomes chronic, cortisol levels stay elevated for too long, and that is when the trouble starts. High cortisol suppresses the immune system, putting it on temporary hold so the body can focus all its energy on dealing with the perceived threat.

This means that during times of stress, our immune cells, the ones that fight off viruses and bacteria, become less active. We are left more vulnerable to infections, slower to heal, and more prone to flare-ups of chronic conditions like cold sores, urinary tract infections, or even autoimmune diseases.

For women, this connection between stress and immunity is especially significant. Our immune systems are already more reactive than men's, in part because of our unique genetic makeup. The X chromosome carries many genes related to immune function, which means women's immune systems are inherently more robust and responsive. But this can be a double-edged sword. On the one hand, it helps us fight off infections more effectively; on the other, it makes us more prone to overactive immune responses, like those seen in autoimmune diseases.

Add chronic stress to the mix, and it is like pouring fuel on a fire. Not only does stress weaken our immune defenses, but it can also trigger or worsen autoimmune flare-ups, creating a vicious cycle of inflammation and illness.

Understanding the link between stress and immunity and how our X chromosome shapes this connection empowers us to take control of our health. By reducing stress and supporting our immune system, we can protect ourselves from illness, recover faster when we do get sick, and create a foundation for long-term well-being.

In the next section, we will see how stress hijacks our cravings, and how the food we eat can create a powerful loop back to worsen or lift our mood. Because what we eat when we are stressed does not just curb our hunger, it is linked to our mental and emotional health.

Stress and Diet

I know how easy it is to reach for comfort foods when stress hits, whether it is a bag of chips, a sugary treat, or that second glass of wine. Trust me, I have been there too. But here is what I have learned: those quick fixes might feel good in the moment, but they can actually make things worse. Processed foods, sugar, and unhealthy fats fuel inflammation in the body, which can worsen anxiety, depression, and even brain fog. It is like pouring gasoline on a fire.

On the flip side, choosing nutrient-dense foods, like leafy greens, fatty fish, nuts, and seeds, can help stabilize your mood, reduce inflammation, and give your brain the fuel it needs to function at its best. I know it is not always easy to make a healthier choice, especially when you are stressed or emotional, but even small changes can make a big difference.

A powerful example of this is the prison study in the UK, where young offenders were given a diet rich in vitamins, minerals, and omega-3s. The results were incredible: violent incidents dropped by 37%, and their behavior and mood improved significantly.[53] This study shows just how much our food choices impact not just our bodies, but our minds and emotions too. So, the next time you are feeling stressed, try reaching for something nourishing instead.

This powerful connection between food and mood reveals an important truth: what we feed our bodies directly shapes our mental resilience. But nutrition is just one piece of the puzzle, because how we move our bodies can be equally transformative for managing stress.

Stress and Exercise

When life feels overwhelming, the last thing you might want to do is exercise. I get it. Some days, just getting off the couch feels like a win. But here's the thing: movement is one of the most powerful tools we must boost our mood and reduce stress. Even a 10-minute walk around the block can release endorphins, those feel-good chemicals that help calm your mind and lift your spirits.

A study published in *The Lancet Psychiatry* found that people who exercised regularly reported 43% fewer days of poor mental health.[54] Activities like team sports, cycling, or even dancing in your living room had the biggest impact. You do not have to run a marathon or spend hours at the gym, just find something you enjoy and move your body. It is not about perfection; it is about showing up for yourself, even in small ways.

Movement helps manage stress, but sleep is what truly restores us. Yet when life gets busy, it is often the first thing we sacrifice. Next, we will discuss why sleep matters.

Stress and Sleep

Ladies, let us talk about sleep. I know how hard it can be to prioritize rest when you are juggling work, family, and a million other responsibilities. But skimping on sleep does not just leave you tired, it messes with your mood, too. Ever experienced feeling irritable and reactive after a poor night's sleep? We all have. Poor sleep disrupts the neurotransmitters that regulate emotions, making you more reactive to stress and more prone to anxiety and depression.

Research from the University of California, Berkeley found that sleep deprivation makes you 60% more reactive to negative emotions.[55] That is a huge shift in how we process stress, and it adds up over time. So, if you are feeling overwhelmed, start with sleep. Create a calming bedtime routine, dim the lights, put away your phone, and give yourself permission to rest.

Sleep heals the body, but connection heals the heart. Just as poor sleep worsens stress, loneliness does too. The good news? Meaningful relationships work with sleep to calm your nervous system.

Stress and Social Connection

As women, we often put everyone else's needs before our own, leaving little time for meaningful connections. Through evolution, women are wired for connection. Those moments of laughter, support, and shared understanding aren't just "nice to have," they are essential for our mental health.

Women are naturally tribal. Many of us maintain friendships from high school to our senior group on the pickle ball court. Unlike the men in our lives, we often cherish these relationships as lifelines, turning to our friend circles not just for fun, but for resilience, healing, and strength.

The *Harvard Study of Adult Development*, which followed people for over 80 years, found that strong social connections are the single biggest predictor of long-term happiness and health.[56] Another study showed that loneliness and social isolation are as harmful to health as smoking 15 cigarettes a day.[57]

So, make time for the people who lift you up, whether it is a phone call with a friend, a coffee date, or even a quick text to say, "*I'm thinking of you.*" You do not have to do it all alone. Connection is your superpower, and investing in your relationships is one of the most healing things you can do.

The Stress Solution

But how do we reduce the effects of stress when life feels like it is constantly throwing challenges at us? This is where Hans Selye's words hit home: *It's not the stress itself that harms us, but how we perceive and react to it.*

Several years ago, while juggling the demands of running a busy medical practice, I felt constantly overwhelmed. I saw stress as something to conquer, something I could outwork, outrun, or ignore. I pushed harder, moved faster, and told myself I could power through it. But that constant state of fight, flight, or freeze took a heavy toll—mentally, physically, and emotionally. It was not the stress breaking me; it was how I was reacting to it.

That is when I met a mindfulness teacher who changed my perspective. He taught me that mindfulness is not about getting rid of stress, it is about changing how we relate to it. Through his guidance, I discovered how mindfulness could help rewire my stress response, calm my nervous system, and build resilience.

We cannot outrun stress, but by shifting our mindset and meeting stress with kindness, compassion, and intentional self-care, we stop reacting from a place of survival and start protecting our health. This shift helps prevent chronic diseases linked to stress and inflammation, like heart disease, diabetes, and autoimmune conditions. When we respond to stress from a place of strength rather than fear, we do not just survive, we thrive. Stress does not have to define us. How we choose to face it can transform us, giving us the power to live healthier, more balanced lives.

While this topic could fill an entire book, I want to share a few simple tools that have made a big difference in my life and can help you, too.

Mindfulness is a powerful tool to build stress resilience. By practicing regularly, you can shift from reacting out of fear to responding from a place of strength, whether you are facing a health challenge, work stress, grief, or relationship troubles.

Stress is a disconnect—a disconnect from our breath, our bodies, our thoughts, and our emotions. Mindfulness is the intentional act of reconnecting to the present moment. It is about using all our senses to observe our physical experiences, thoughts, and emotions with curiosity and full acceptance. It is not about trying to change the experience; it is simply about being aware of it, exactly as it is.

This reconnection can happen through formal practices or informal moments woven into daily life. Here are some powerful mindfulness tools that can help you reconnect with your body, calm your nervous system, and build resilience:

Formal Mindfulness Practices

These exercises are simple tools to train your attention. You do not need anything special, just a few minutes and a willingness to notice. Start with just 2-3 minutes. When your mind wanders (which it will!), softly bring it back. That is all there is to it.

1. Body Scan

Lie down or sit comfortably and slowly bring your attention to each part of your body, from your toes to your head. Simply notice sensations without judgment.

Tool: Use this practice to release tension and reconnect with your body, especially before bed or after a long day.

2. Sitting Meditation

Sit quietly, focus on your breath, and observe your thoughts as they arise and pass, without getting caught up in them.

Tool: Start with 5-10 minutes daily to build awareness and calm your mind.

3. Breath Practice

Pause and take a few deep breaths, focusing on the sensation of air moving in and out of your lungs.

Tool: Try the 4-7-8 technique (inhale for 4, hold for 7, exhale for 8) to instantly calm your nervous system.

4. Five Senses

Pause and notice one thing you can see, hear, touch, taste, and smell.

Tool: Use this to ground yourself during moments of overwhelm.

5. Mindful Movement

Practice gentle yoga, stretching, or walking while paying attention to how your body feels.

Tool: Move slowly and intentionally to release stress and improve focus.

6. Journaling

Write freely about your thoughts, emotions, or experiences without judgment.

Tool: Use prompts like *"What am I feeling right now?"* to process emotions and gain clarity.

7. Guided Imagery

Close your eyes and visualize a peaceful place, such as a beach, forest, or your favorite cozy space.

Tool: Use this visualization to reduce anxiety and create a sense of calm.

8. Progressive Muscle Relaxation

Tense and release each muscle group, beginning at your toes and working your way up to your head.

Tool: Use this technique to relieve physical tension and promote relaxation.

9. Body Tapping

Gently tap different parts of your body like your shoulders, arms, or chest. Tapping can help calm your mind, ease stress, and bring quick relief when you are feeling.

Tool: This can help release emotional blockages and re-energize your body.

Informal Mindfulness Practices in Daily Life

Mindfulness is not limited to a meditation cushion; it can be woven into the everyday movements of life. These informal practices help bring you back to the present, even in the middle of a busy day.

1. Mindful Eating

Slow down and savor each bite, noticing the taste, texture, and aroma of your food.

Tool: Use this to improve digestion, reduce stress-related overeating, and reconnect with the joy of nourishing your body.

2. Mindful Communication

Listen actively during conversations, pause before responding, and stay fully present.

Tool: This reduces misunderstandings and helps you respond with intention rather than reactivity.

3. Mindful Driving

Notice the feeling of your hands on the wheel, the sound of the engine, and the rhythm of your breath.

Tool: Turn your commute into a peaceful pause rather than a stress trigger.

Building a Mindfulness Habit

You do not have to be perfect; you just have to begin. Like any habit, mindfulness becomes more natural the more you practice. Here's how to build a habit that sticks:

1. Start Small

Dedicate just five minutes a day to mindfulness. Anchor your practice to existing habits, like brushing your teeth, waiting for your coffee to brew, or putting on your shoes.

Tool: Small, consistent steps make mindfulness sustainable.

2. Create a Routine

Try morning meditation, a midday breathing break, or an evening body scan to unwind.

Tool: Consistency matters more than duration. Find what fits your lifestyle and let it become your rhythm.

3. Overcome Challenges

It is normal to feel restless or distracted at first. Be kind to yourself, this is part of the process. Use guided meditations or apps to stay on track.

Tool: Remember, mindfulness is practice, not performance. Progress is what matters most.

By weaving both formal and informal mindfulness into your life, you can transform your relationship with stress. It is not about eliminating every challenge, it is about meeting each moment with compassion, awareness, and strength. That is where true resilience is built.

Suggested Supplements for Mental Health

Always consult your healthcare provider before starting any new supplement. And remember, supplements are never a replacement for professional mental health support. See Appendix B for a list of these recommended supplements for mental health.

Final Thoughts

I know firsthand how overwhelming stress can feel. But stress does not have to define you.

By practicing mindfulness, even in small ways like pausing to breathe or savoring a meal, you can start to shift from reacting out of fear to responding from a place of strength.

Mindfulness is not about perfection. It is about full acceptance of where we are in the process, starting awareness of the perception of stress. Then bring attention to your breath, body, thoughts, and feelings. Each check-in creates space for tiny shifts that guide your next steps.

Start small, be kind to yourself. Trust that the small steps matter. You have the power to transform your relationship with stress and create a life that feels balanced, resilient, and full of possibility.

Questions to Discuss With Your Doctor:

These questions are designed to help you have a more informed, collaborative conversation with your healthcare provider, so you can get to the root of what is going on and build a plan that supports your mental, emotional, and physical well-being.

1. Could my mood symptoms (fatigue, anxiety, mood swings) be linked to underlying medical conditions?

Consider: Thyroid dysfunction, hormonal imbalances, or metabolic issues. Request testing for a full hormone panel, thyroid panel (TSH, free T3, free T4, reverse T3, thyroid antibodies), timed salivary cortisol, micronutrient testing, and inflammation markers like hs-CRP or IL-6.

2. Could my gut health be impacting my mental health?

Discuss: Stool microbiome testing to assess gut dysbiosis, leaky gut markers, and microbiome diversity, as gut health is closely linked to brain health.

3. Could food sensitivities or allergies be contributing to my symptoms?

Consider: Food sensitivity testing or an elimination diet to identify potential triggers like gluten, dairy, or other allergens.

4. Could nutrient deficiencies or genetic factors play a role?

Request: Micronutrient testing, organic acid testing, and genetic SNP testing for variants like MTHFR or COMT, which can impact neurotransmitter production and stress response.

5. Could toxins like heavy metals be affecting my mental health?

Consider: Heavy metal testing to rule out exposure to toxins like lead, mercury, or arsenic, which can impact brain function.

6. Could my medical conditions (e.g., blood pressure, hormonal imbalances, gut issues) be linked to my stress levels?

Discuss: How chronic stress might be exacerbating your symptoms and explore strategies to address it.

7. Are there non-pharmaceutical options that could support my mental health?

Consider: Supplements like omega-3 fatty acids, magnesium, B vitamins, adaptogens (e.g., ashwagandha, rhodiola), or therapies like cognitive behavioral therapy (CBT), mindfulness, or acupuncture.

8. What lifestyle changes do you recommend to help me manage stress and build resilience?

Discuss: Dietary changes like an anti-inflammatory or Mediterranean diet, regular exercise, stress management techniques (e.g., meditation, yoga, deep breathing), and sleep hygiene practices.

9. Can we evaluate my sleep patterns, as poor sleep can worsen mental health?

Consider: Sleep testing or referrals to a sleep specialist if issues like insomnia or sleep apnea are suspected.

10. Can you refer me to specialists who can help me further?

Consider: A nutritionist for dietary guidance, a therapist for mental health support, or an integrative medicine practitioner for a comprehensive approach.

11. Can we partner together to create a preventative health plan for my mental well-being?

Work with your doctor to develop a personalized plan that addresses your unique needs, symptoms, and goals.

For a complete companion resource, including all "Questions to Discuss with Your Doctor," Supplement Lists, and Guides, scan the QR code.

Chapter 6

Immune Health

"The human immune system is a double-edged sword."

—**Jeffrey S. Bland, PhD**

Have you ever heard of the so-called "man-cold"? I recently came across a social media reel that perfectly illustrated this phenomenon. In it, a woman with the flu is shown powering through her day. She is working, cleaning the house, grocery shopping, and taking care of her children, while feeling under the weather. Then the scene cuts to her husband, who has the same flu, and he's completely bedridden, surrounded by a fortress of tissues, utterly incapacitated. Sound familiar?

While it is easy to laugh at this stereotype, it highlights an important truth: women and men often experience infections and immune responses very differently. As a doctor, I find this fascinating, and as a woman, I think it is something we should all be aware of. Research shows that women's immune systems tend to be more reactive and robust compared to men's. This can be both a blessing and a challenge. On the one hand, it may mean we recover more quickly from illnesses like colds or the flu. On the other hand, this heightened immune response can make us more susceptible to autoimmune diseases, where the immune system mistakenly attacks the body it is designed to protect. In a way, our immune system is both our greatest ally and, at times, our own toughest opponent.

Men, by contrast, often have a less reactive immune system. While this might mean they take longer to bounce back from infections, it also makes them less prone to autoimmune conditions. These differences are rooted in biology, hormones, genetics, and even the way our immune cells communicate play a role.

As women, our immune systems are incredibly complex and powerful, but they also require extra care and attention to stay in balance. Understanding these nuances is not just a matter of curiosity, it is crucial that doctors provide women with timely, personalized care. When it comes to our bodies, one size definitely does not fit all.

A Patient Story: Sarah's Journey

In my medical practice, I have seen time and again how female patients present with intricate and interconnected immune system challenges. Let me share the story of Sarah, a vibrant 47-year-old woman who came to me after dealing with a serious health issue. Sarah had always been the picture of health, until she caught a cold. She developed a dry cough, low-grade fever, body aches, and fatigue. She thought it might be a mild case of the flu, which was later confirmed to be COVID-19 by a PCR test. She rested at home, and after five days, the flu-like symptoms began to ease. She thought she was in the clear.

But then, a week later, Sarah's body sent her a clear and alarming message that something was wrong. She woke up in the middle of the night with her heart racing, drenched in sweat, and gasping for air. Her hands trembled, her mood was erratic, and sleep became a distant memory. Her body felt like it was stuck in overdrive, and she knew something was seriously wrong.

At the emergency department, Sarah's blood pressure was dangerously high, and her heart rate was through the roof. Blood tests revealed her thyroid was in overdrive. Further testing confirmed she had Graves' disease, an autoimmune condition where the immune system attacks the thyroid, causing it to go into hyperdrive. She was told her condition was genetic and was given the standard medical options: medication or radiation treatment that would shut down her thyroid gland permanently.

Sarah was stunned. This had come out of nowhere. Why had this happened to her? Could she recover without aggressive medical interventions? She was searching for a different path, one that would address the root cause and restore balance to her immune system.

I explained to Sarah that genes load the gun, but it is our lifestyle, environment, food choices, exposure to pollutants, infections and chronic psychosocial stress that fire the bullets. And just as those genes get turned on by a trigger, they can be turned off by addressing the root cause.

But most importantly, we focused on hope and action. Though most autoimmune diseases are chronic and without a cure, the goal is to alleviate symptoms, control future tissue damage, and work toward remission. Together, we created a plan to restore balance by supporting her immune system, healing her gut, reducing inflammation, and addressing the stressors in her life.

Sarah's journey is a reminder that while autoimmune conditions can feel overwhelming, there are ways to take back control and work toward remission. It is not always easy, but with the right tools and support, it is possible to find balance and reclaim your health.

Let us take a closer look at how the immune system works and how we can support it in a way that works for you.

When Our Immune System Turns Against Us

If you are like me, you have probably wondered, *why did this happen to me?* The truth is, we do not have all the answers yet, but we do know that autoimmune diseases are often the result of a perfect storm—genetics, gut issues, environmental triggers, infections, and lifestyle factors all play a role. Let us break it down so you can understand what might be going on in your body or the body of someone you love.

Your immune system is like your body's personal military, a highly trained defense force designed to protect you. To fulfil its mission, the immune system must be able to tell the difference between your own cells (the good guys) and harmful invaders like bacteria, viruses, or toxins (the bad guys). This ability to recognize you is called *self-tolerance*.

But sometimes, something in your environment, like an infection, a toxin, or chronic stress, can accidentally flip the wrong switch in your immune system's command center. Suddenly, your military loses its ability to recognize you. It starts seeing your own tissues as the enemy and launches an attack. This friendly fire is what we call *autoimmunity*, and it is how autoimmune diseases begin.

Certain viruses and bacteria, like Epstein-Barr virus (EBV), cytomegalovirus (CMV), and even COVID-19, have been linked to autoimmune diseases. One theory is that these pathogens confuse your immune system through a process called *molecular mimicry*—they look so similar to your own tissues that your immune system starts attacking both the invader and your own cells.

Women are far more likely than men to develop autoimmune diseases, yet in medicine, we often do not look for the root cause. Instead, doctors tend to focus on the specific organ or area under attack, like the thyroid in Graves' disease or Hashimoto's, the joints in rheumatoid arthritis, or the skin in lupus, vitiligo, or psoriasis. You might think you have a thyroid issue, a joint issue, or a skin issue, but here's the truth: those organs are innocent bystanders caught in the crossfire. The real problem is a dysregulated immune system.

Think of it like a fire. When your immune system misfires, it is like a spark that ignites inflammation in one part of your body. If we do not address what is fueling the fire, it does not stay contained. It spreads. This is why so many patients with one autoimmune disease end up developing another. Without treating the underlying issue, the fire keeps burning, moving from one area to the next.

Over 80 different conditions fall under the autoimmune umbrella, from lupus and rheumatoid arthritis to Crohn's disease and type 1 diabetes. Together, they affect more than 24 million people in the U.S. and one in ten people worldwide. And here's the kicker: 80% of all autoimmune cases are in women.[58] If you are reading this, chances are you or someone you love has felt the weight of these diseases.

The result? Inflammation, pain, and damage, a body literally at war with itself. It is time to stop just putting out the flames in one area and start addressing the fire at its source. Because when we do, we can help your body heal and prevent the fire from spreading.

Up next, let us explore your gut, which acts as the command center for your immune system and can either fuel the fire or help extinguish it.

The Gut-Immune Connection: Where It All Begins

Did you know that 70% of your immune system lives in your gut?[59] Your gut microbiome, the trillions of bacteria living in your digestive tract, plays a huge role in regulating your immune system.

Your gut microbiome is like a bustling city, with good bacteria (the "good guys") and bad bacteria (the "troublemakers"). When the balance is right, the good guys keep the troublemakers in check, and your immune system stays calm. But when the balance is disrupted, by a diet high in sugar, processed foods, or antibiotics, the troublemakers can take over. This can lead to a condition called *leaky gut*, where the lining of your intestines becomes more permeable, allowing toxins and undigested food particles to leak into your bloodstream. Your immune system sees these invaders and sounds the alarm, leading to chronic inflammation and, over time, autoimmune disease.

In modern medicine, we excel at rescuing patients from acute autoimmune attacks using medications and immunosuppressants to prevent tissue and organ damage, and this is often necessary and lifesaving. But while we manage symptoms, we often overlook the root cause: Why is the immune system misfiring in the first place? What if, instead of just managing symptoms, we worked to calm the immune system, reduce inflammation, and uncover the root cause?

That is the approach I believe in, one that does not just treat the problem but helps you heal from within. It is about retaining the immune system by healing your gut, reducing toxins, calming inflammation, and managing stress. We do this using anti-inflammatory foods, mind-body practices, and personalized nutrition to address root causes.

So where do we start? In the next section, I will guide you through step-by-step changes you can make to begin healing your immune system from the inside out.

Food and Autoimmunity: Healing Through What You Eat

Now that we have explored the gut-immune connection, let us talk about one of the most powerful tools you have to support your immune system, your diet.

When Sarah came to me, she was struggling with Graves' disease, an autoimmune condition that had turned her life upside down. She was exhausted, anxious, and frustrated, her body felt like it was betraying her. One of the first things we worked on together was her diet. Why? Because what you eat can either fuel inflammation or help calm it down. For Sarah, making changes to her diet became a game-changer.

The Autoimmune Protocol (AIP): A Reset for Your Immune System

The Autoimmune Protocol, or AIP, is like a reset button. It works for many patients by calming the immune system and giving the body space to heal. It is designed to remove foods that commonly trigger inflammation and immune reactions for a short period of time, offering your immune system a break. Here's how it works:

What You Eliminate:

- **Grains**: Especially gluten-containing grains like wheat, barley, and rye.
- **Dairy**: All forms, including milk, cheese, and yogurt.
- **Legumes**: Beans, lentils, peanuts, and soy.
- **Nightshades**: Tomatoes, potatoes, eggplants, and peppers.
- **Processed Foods:** Anything with artificial additives, preservatives, or refined sugars.
- **Eggs, Nuts, and Seeds:** These are also removed initially, as they can be inflammatory for some people.

What You Focus On:

- Vegetables: Especially leafy greens, cruciferous veggies (like broccoli and cauliflower), and colorful options like carrots and beets.
- Clean Proteins: Grass-fed meats, wild-caught fish, and organ meats (rich in nutrients).
- Healthy Fats: Avocado, coconut oil, and olive oil.
- Fruits: In moderation, focusing on low-sugar options like berries.
- Healing Foods: Bone broth, fermented foods (like sauerkraut), and herbs like turmeric and ginger.

Reintroducing Foods:

After 4-6 weeks (or longer, depending on how you feel), you slowly reintroduce eliminated foods, one at a time. This helps you identify which foods might be triggering your symptoms. For example, Sarah discovered that dairy and gluten caused bloating and fatigue, so she decided to avoid them long-term.

The Wahls Protocol: Feeding Your Cells

Another powerful approach is the Wahls Protocol, created by Dr. Terry Wahls, a physician who improved her own multiple sclerosis symptoms through diet and lifestyle changes. This protocol focuses on nourishing your mitochondria, the energy powerhouses in your cells, to support overall health and reduce inflammation.[60]

The Science Behind It:

Mitochondria need specific nutrients to function properly, like B vitamins, antioxidants, and omega-3 fatty acids. When they are damaged or undernourished, it can lead to fatigue, brain fog, and inflammation.

The Wahls Protocol emphasizes eating nine cups of vegetables and fruit each day, divided into three nutrient-rich categories:

1. **Leafy Greens:** Spinach, kale, and Swiss chard for vitamins and minerals.
2. **Colorful Fruits and Veggies:** Berries, carrots, and beets for antioxidants.
3. **Sulfur-Rich Vegetables:** Broccoli, cauliflower, garlic, and onions for detox support.

It also includes high-quality proteins, organ meats, and healthy fats to support cell repair and energy production.

By flooding your body with nutrient-dense foods, the Wahls Protocol helps repair cellular damage, reduce inflammation, and support your immune system. Many of my patients, including Sarah, have found that combining elements of AIP and Wahls, like focusing on vegetables and clean proteins, helps them feel their best.

Why These Diets Work

Both AIP and Wahls are rooted in science. They reduce inflammation by removing common dietary triggers while flooding your body with the nutrients it needs to heal. For Sarah, cutting out gluten and dairy while adding more vegetables and healthy fats made a noticeable difference in her energy levels and overall well-being.

The key takeaway? Food is powerful medicine. By making intentional choices about what you eat, you can calm your immune system, reduce inflammation, and take control of your health. This may be challenging to do alone, seek out professional help with a functional nutritionist or doctor who can help guide you.

Environmental Exposures: Practical Solutions to Reduce Toxins

Let us talk about the world we live in, because it is changing, and not always for the better. Autoimmune diseases are on the rise, and it is no coincidence. The quality of our food has declined, filled with additives, chemicals, and antibiotics. We are exposed to heavy metals like mercury, pesticides in our produce, air pollution in our cities, and even chemicals used in dry cleaning. These exposures can quietly overload our system, and over time increase the risk of developing an autoimmune disease.

These toxins create something called oxidative stress in your body. Think of it like rust forming on metal that gradually damages your cells and tissues. This is especially hard on your mitochondria, the tiny powerhouses in your cells that produce energy. When mitochondria are damaged, they cannot function properly, leading to fatigue, inflammation, and a confused immune system. The result? A body that is tired, inflamed and more likely to turn against itself. Over time, this oxidative stress can trigger chronic inflammation and make your immune system more likely to misfire and attack your own body.

Let us next look at practical ways to reduce your toxic load and support your body's natural detox systems, because knowledge is power, and small changes can make a big impact.

Water: Clean Hydration for a Healthy Body

The water you drink can also impact your health. Tap water often contains chemicals like chlorine, fluoride, and even traces of heavy metals. To ensure your water is clean and safe, consider investing in a high-quality water filter. Drinking plenty of clean water helps flush out toxins, supports your immune system,

Air: Breathe Easier with Clean Indoor Air

Air pollution can affect your lungs, and it can impact your immune system. Pollutants like car exhaust, industrial chemicals, and even mold spores in your home can trigger inflammation and oxidative stress. To improve your air quality, try adding indoor plants like spider plants, peace lilies, and snake plants, which naturally filter toxins. On days when air pollution is high, keep your windows closed, and consider investing in an air purifier with a HEPA filter to keep your indoor air clean.

Household Products: Swap Toxins for Clean Alternatives

Many common cleaning products, laundry detergents, and even candles contain harmful chemicals like phthalates, parabens, and volatile organic compounds (VOCs). To reduce your exposure, switch to natural, non-toxic cleaning alternatives. You can even make your own cleaners with vinegar, baking soda and essential oils. Look for products labeled 'fragrance-free' or 'non-toxic' to avoid harmful chemicals.

Beauty and Skin Products: Protect Your Skin, Protect Your Health

Your skin is your body's largest organ, and what you put on it gets absorbed into your bloodstream. Many beauty and skincare products contain synthetic fragrances, preservatives, and other chemicals that can trigger immune reactions. Use apps like Yuka (yuka.io) or Think Dirty (thinkdirtyapp.com) to scan product barcodes in the store before you buy them to check ingredients and safety ratings.

What you eat, drink, breathe, and put on your body all play a role in your immune health. By making small, mindful changes in these areas, you can reduce your toxic load, calm inflammation, and support your body's natural ability to heal and protect. While reducing your exposure to toxins helps strengthen your immune system, there's another invisible threat that can undermine your efforts: stress.

Stress: The Silent Immune Saboteur

Okay, let us get real about stress for a minute. We have all been there—feeling overwhelmed, exhausted, and like we are running on empty. Maybe you remember getting frequent colds during finals week or always catching everything at the office when you were working long hours on a project. Sound familiar? That is because stress does not just leave you feeling drained, it weakens your immune system, making you more vulnerable to infections like colds, flu, or even recurrent sinus issues.

Here's why that happens: when you are stressed, your body releases cortisol, a hormone designed to help you handle short-term challenges. In moderation, cortisol is helpful. But when stress becomes chronic, that cortisol keeps firing, suppressing parts of your immune system and reducing your body's ability to fight off germs and viruses.

But here's the twist, stress does not just swing the pendulum in one direction. At the same time, it is weakening your immune defenses, it can over activate other parts of your immune system, ramping up inflammation and triggering autoimmune flares. It is like your immune system is stuck in a tug-of-war, and stress is pulling the rope from both ends. This double whammy can leave you feeling exhausted, unwell, and stuck in a cycle of infections and autoimmune flare-ups.

Here are some practical, science-backed strategies for building habits that help your body handle stress better.

1. Prioritize Good Sleep Practices

Sleep is your body's time to repair and recharge, and it is essential for keeping your immune system strong. Poor sleep can increase cortisol levels and leave you more vulnerable to stress and inflammation. Here's how to improve your sleep:

- **Stick to a Schedule:** Go to bed and wake up at the same time every day, even on weekends.
- **Create a Relaxing Routine:** Wind down with calming activities like reading, taking a warm bath, or practicing gentle yoga.
- **Limit Screen Time:** Avoid phones, tablets, and TVs at least an hour before bed, the blue light can disrupt your sleep.
- **Optimize Your Sleep Environment:** Keep your bedroom cool, dark, and quiet, and invest in a comfortable mattress and pillows.

2. Move Your Body (But Do not Overdo It)

Exercise is one of the best ways to reduce stress and support your immune system. It lowers cortisol levels, boosts endorphins (your body's natural mood lifters), and improves circulation, helping immune cells move through your body more effectively. Here's how to make it work for you:

- **Find What You Enjoy**: Whether it is walking, dancing, yoga, or swimming, choose activities that feel good and fit your lifestyle.
- **Keep It Moderate**: Over-exercising can increase stress on your body, so aim for a balance that leaves you energized, not exhausted.
- **Get Outside**: Spending time in nature can reduce stress and boost your mood.

3. Cultivate Social Connections

Humans are wired for connection. Strong relationships can be a powerful buffer against stress. Studies show that people with strong social support have better immune function and lower levels of inflammation. Here's how to nurture your connections:

- **Reach Out:** Make time for friends and family, even just a quick phone call or text.
- **Join a Community:** Whether it is a book club, fitness class, or support group, being part of a community can help you feel less alone.
- **Practice Gratitude:** Let the people in your life know you appreciate them. It strengthens your bonds and boosts your mood.

4. Practice Mind-Body Techniques

Mind-body practices are a game-changer for managing stress and calming your immune system. They help lower cortisol levels, reduce inflammation, and bring your nervous system back into balance. Try one or more of these:

- **Meditation**: Even 5-10 minutes a day can make a difference. Apps like Insight Timer or Headspace can help you get started.
- **Deep Breathing**: Try belly breathing or the 4-7-8 method for deep relaxation.

- **Yoga or Tai Chi**: These practices combine movement with mindfulness, helping you release tension and stay grounded.
- **Journaling**: Writing down your thoughts and feelings can help you process stress and gain perspective.

By addressing the root causes of stress, supporting your gut health, and reducing your exposure to toxins, you can calm your immune system, reduce inflammation, and take control of your health.

And remember, you are not just a collection of symptoms. You are a whole person, and you deserve care that honors your full story.

Suggested Supplements for Immune Health

Supplements can be a helpful addition to your wellness toolkit, especially when paired with a healthy lifestyle and personalized care. Whether you are trying to support your immune system during cold and flu season or manage autoimmune conditions, these evidence-based options can offer extra support. As always, consult your healthcare provider before starting any new supplement, especially if you are managing an autoimmune condition or taking medications. See Appendix B for a list of these recommended supplements for immune health.

Final Thoughts

When it comes to immune health, women face unique challenges. Our immune systems are more reactive by design, which can be both a strength and a vulnerability. But here's the good news: we have the power to influence our health.

By focusing on a nutrient-rich diet, managing stress, prioritizing sleep, and reducing toxin exposure, we can create an internal environment that supports our immune systems and lowers the risk of both infections and autoimmune flare-ups.

Remember, your health is a journey. And every small step you take, every nourishing choice, every moment of rest, and every boundary you set matters. When we support our immune system from the inside out, we are not just reacting to illness, we are proactively building resilience, vitality, and long-term well-being.

Questions To Discuss With Your Doctor:

These questions are designed to help you have a more informed, collaborative conversation with your healthcare provider, so you can get to the root of what is going on and build a plan that supports your mental, emotional, and physical well-being.

1. Can I get lab work to assess my immune health?

Consider: Comprehensive metabolic panel (CMP), complete blood count (CBC), thyroid panel, vitamin D3, zinc, selenium, hs-CRP, ESR, ANA, anti-dsDNA, thyroid antibodies, AVISE® CTD autoimmune panel, food sensitivity testing, gut microbiome analysis, and heavy metal testing.

2. Would testing for infections like Epstein-Barr virus (EBV), cytomegalovirus (CMV), or Lyme disease be helpful?

These infections can trigger or exacerbate autoimmune conditions.

3. Can we explore my gut health?

Consider: Stool testing for dysbiosis, leaky gut markers, and microbiome diversity.

4. Are there any vitamins or supplements that could support my immune health?

Consider: Vitamin D3, omega-3 fatty acids, probiotics, curcumin, N-acetylcysteine (NAC), quercetin, and zinc.

5. Can we test for nutrient deficiencies that might be impacting my immune system?

Consider: Vitamin D, B vitamins, magnesium, zinc, and selenium.

6. Can we create a plan to reduce my exposure to environmental toxins?

Discuss: Testing for heavy metals, mold exposure, and strategies to minimize toxins in your home, diet, and personal care products.

7. Are there lifestyle changes we can focus on to support my immune system?

Discuss: Stress management techniques, sleep optimization, exercise, and dietary changes like an anti-inflammatory or autoimmune protocol (AIP) diet.

8. Can we partner together to create a preventative health plan for my immune system?

Work with your doctor to develop a personalized plan that addresses your unique needs and goals.

For a complete companion resource, including all "Questions to Discuss with Your Doctor," Supplement Lists, and Guides, scan the QR code.

Chapter 7

Digestive Health

"All disease begins in the gut."

—Hippocrates

It is remarkable how much modern medicine has advanced, yet how little we, as doctors, talk to you, our patients, about food, nutrition, and digestion. Hippocrates' timeless wisdom reminds us that the gut is the foundation of well-being, but in medical school, this truth often gets overlooked. I spent years learning to diagnose and treat diseases, but I was rarely taught how to prevent illness using food. Even more surprising? I was not taught about the profound differences between men and women when it comes to digestive health, from the anatomy of our intestines to how they function and even the unique struggles we, as women, are more likely to face. Did you know that your small intestines as a woman are 30 cm longer and your colon is 10 cm longer than a man's?[61]

No wonder we have differences in our bowel habits! Maybe you can relate to my little story about my husband's morning routine. Every single day at 8 a.m., like clockwork, he heads to the bathroom, spends a few minutes, and emerges like it is no big deal. No fuss, no drama. Meanwhile, for me and maybe for many of you, it is not always that simple. Sometimes it is days before things move, and when they do, it is often with constipation, diarrhea, discomfort, or bloating. Sound familiar?

So, why is there such a big difference between men and women when it comes to digestion? As a doctor, I can tell you—it all comes down to biology. Men tend to have shorter, straighter intestines, which means food moves through their system more quickly and efficiently. For us women, it is a different story. Our intestines are longer, narrower, and more winding, which can slow things down and make us more prone to constipation, especially during times of stress or hormonal shifts like PMS, pregnancy, or menopause.

But that is not all. We, women, also have a more sensitive Vagus nerve and enteric nervous system (often called the "gut brain"), which means our digestion is more easily influenced by mental, emotional, and physical stress. On top of that, our gut microbiome, the community of bacteria living in our digestive tract, is different from men's. This microbiome plays a huge role in how we process food, absorb nutrients, and even manage mood. Research shows that hormonal fluctuations can directly impact the balance of our gut bacteria, which may explain why we often experience more digestive ups and downs. Add to that unique problems we can develop, like uterine fibroids, pelvic inflammation during our periods or pelvic organ prolapse, which can put extra pressure on the intestines and further complicate things. And let us not forget how factors like travel, jet lag, and even certain foods can throw our digestive systems completely off balance.

All these symptoms are often given a "catch-all" diagnosis called Irritable Bowel Syndrome (IBS), a condition that affects women at nearly twice the rate of men.[62] IBS includes a wide range of symptoms which include bloating, cramping, diarrhea, constipation, or a mix of both, without a clear underlying cause. While it is one of the most common digestive disorders, there is still a lot we do not know about why it is so much more prevalent in women. Unfortunately, there is a lack of research focused specifically on women's digestive health, which means many of us are left navigating these issues without clear answers or tailored solutions.

This gap in understanding leaves many doctors unprepared to address your gut issues beyond a referral for a colonoscopy or a prescription of antacids. But here is what you need to know: the gut does not just digest food, it influences everything from mood to heart health, brain health, and immunity. And our digestive health is deeply tied to what we eat, how we live, and even our gender.

If you have ever felt like your gut symptoms weren't taken seriously or dismissed as "normal," you are not alone. Let us look at how this plays out in real life with a patient story that may sound a lot like your own.

A Patient Story: Mona's Journey

Let me share Mona's story with you. Mona was a 59-year-old woman who had been diagnosed with irritable bowel syndrome (IBS) years ago after struggling with persistent gas and bloating. She couldn't remember the last time she felt "normal". It had been over a decade since she had a flat stomach or could eat without worrying about the consequences. These days, nearly every meal left her with a distended "food belly" that could take days to settle. Frustrated and exhausted by her health struggles, she decided to explore an integrative approach to healing. That is when our paths crossed.

Mona opened up about her life as a single parent to twin boys. Over the past decade, she had worked tirelessly to provide for her family, especially to send her sons to college. But the stress of it all had taken a toll. She had been laid off from her job at one point and struggled to find stability until she eventually secured another position. However, the constant financial and work-related stress pushed her to her breaking point. She began experiencing panic attacks, anxiety, and worsening digestive symptoms. To cope with the bloating that followed every meal, she started wearing loose clothing, hoping to hide her discomfort. Over the years, she also dealt with recurring skin infections, which led to multiple rounds of antibiotics.

We ran a series of labs, which revealed significantly elevated inflammation markers, including an hs-CRP that was 9 times higher than normal. This confirmed that her body was under considerable stress. We also identified moderate to severe food sensitivities and developed a personalized elimination plan to give her gut a chance to heal. Interestingly, her SIBO (small intestine bacterial overgrowth) test came back normal, ruling out a common culprit for IBS. However, her stool test told a more complex story. It was positive for both *H. pylori* and *Giardia*, two infections that can wreak havoc on the digestive system. Additionally, the test showed poor pancreatic function, and dysbiosis, an imbalance in her gut microbiome with overgrowths of *Staph*, *Strep*, methane-producing *Methanobacteriaceae*, and inflammation-triggering Citrobacter.

To address these findings, we took a multi-layered approach. We treated the infections with targeted therapies, supported her digestion with enzymes, and introduced probiotics to help restore balance. We also focused on rebuilding her gut microbiome through fermented foods, prebiotic fibers, resistance starches, polyphenols, and short-chain fatty acids. Recognizing the profound connection between her gut and brain, we incorporated stress resilience practices into her routine. She began daily meditation and breathwork to improve vagal tone, which helps regulate the nervous system. She also started using the Nerva app, an evidence-based gut-directed hypnotherapy program designed to enhance communication between the gut and brain.

We worked together to create a daily rhythm that prioritized stability and grounding. Her days began and ended with mindful practices, and she followed a structured schedule with regular mealtimes and consistent bedtimes. This routine helped her feel more in control and less reactive to the stressors in her life.

Over time, Mona's symptoms began to improve. She could reintroduce the foods she had eliminated slowly, and her bloating and discomfort diminished. But perhaps the most profound shift came from her own self-reflection. Through this journey, Mona discovered a desire to help others navigate their challenges. She decided to pivot her career and pursue life coaching, taking steps toward a path that brought her purpose and joy.

Mona's story is one I hear all too often in my practice. It is a reminder of how deeply interconnected our physical health, emotional well-being, and lifestyle stressors can be. Her journey also highlights the importance of addressing health challenges holistically, considering not just the symptoms but the whole person—mind, body, and life circumstances. Together, we began to unravel the layers of her condition, working toward a path of healing that honored her unique needs and experiences.

In the next section, we will explore how your thoughts, emotions, and stress levels directly influence your digestion, and what you can do to create healthier gut-brain communication.

Digestion Starts in the Mind

You might think digestion is food goes in, gets broken down, nutrients are absorbed, and waste is eliminated. But the truth is, digestion is deeply influenced by your mental, emotional, and even spiritual state.

Digestion is not just about what you eat, it is about how you eat, where your food comes from, the mindset you are in when you prepare it, who you eat with, and even the distractions around you while you eat. All these factors affect your digestion through your gut-brain axis.

When you eat a meal, you have lovingly prepared, sitting at a table with people you care about, savoring each bite without distractions, your body is in a state of calm. Your parasympathetic nervous system, the "rest and digest" mode, activates the Vagus nerve, allowing your digestive system to work efficiently. But when you are rushing through a meal, eating while stressed, at your desk at work or scrolling through your phone, your body shifts into "fight or flight" mode. Energy is diverted away from digestion, leading to slowed motility, bloating, and even nutrient malabsorption.

For us women, this connection is even more pronounced. Our more sensitive nervous systems and hormonal fluctuations mean that stress, anxiety, and emotional upheaval can hit our digestion harder. That is why practices like mindfulness, meditation, and breathwork are essential tools for calming the nervous system and allowing your gut to function at its best. Consider the Nerva app (nervahealth.com), as Mona did, it is designed to help balance the gut-brain axis through vagal toning. By incorporating mindfulness and stress-resilience practices into her daily routine, she was able to calm her nervous system and ultimately heal her gut.

So, the next time you sit down to eat, take a moment to pause. Consider where your food came from, the love and intention that went into preparing it, and the environment you are eating in. Are you distracted? Stressed? Rushing? Or are you present, calm, and grateful for the nourishment in front of you? These small mindset shifts can have a profound impact on your digestion and your overall well-being.

Digestion: The Path Food Takes

Let us also talk about the incredible journey your food takes from the moment it enters your mouth to when it leaves your body. Think of it like a well-planned road trip, where every stop along the way is crucial to reaching the final destination. If something goes wrong at any point, the whole trip can get derailed. So, let us walk through this journey together, step by step, so you can understand how it all works and what can go wrong.

Digestion starts in your mouth. Chewing breaks food into smaller pieces, and enzymes in your saliva begin breaking it down, this is the first crucial step in the digestive process. But your mouth is also home to its own microbiome. If you do not chew properly, eat too quickly, or suffer from dry mouth, you are sabotaging this vital stage. A healthy oral microbiome not only supports digestion but also helps protect against gum disease, bad breath, and even systemic inflammation.

From there, your food travels down the esophagus, a muscular tube that acts like a conveyor belt moving everything toward your stomach. This process is powered by the Vagus nerve, which can be thrown off by stress. If the esophagus narrows, is infected with candida, injured by acid or does not function properly, you might experience food getting stuck, pain, or trouble swallowing. Stress can make things worse, as it weakens the Vagus nerve's ability to keep things moving smoothly, sometimes causing food and stomach acid to flow back up into the esophagus, leading to acid reflux.

Once your food reaches the stomach, gastric acid and enzymes continue breaking it down into usable nutrients. But imbalances due to H. pylori infections, low stomach acid from chronic stress (often due to aging, antibiotics, or antacids), or a weak valve allowing food to reflux into the esophagus can lead to ulcers, gastritis, or acid reflux. The stomach is also responsible for secretion of appetite regulating hormones like ghrelin, which can affect hunger and cravings, leading to weight gain.

Next stop: the small intestine. Imagine it like a car wash: finger-like projections on the lining of the small intestine move the food along while it gets sprayed with bile from your liver and enzymes from your pancreas and gut lining. These help break down fats, proteins, and carbohydrates into their smallest components, which are then absorbed into your bloodstream to fuel your body. An overgrowth of bacteria in the small intestine, called SIBO (often triggered by antibiotics, antacids, stress, or toxins), can cause gas, bloating, constipation, diarrhea, malabsorption, and abdominal pain. If your pancreas, liver, or gallbladder are not functioning well, these symptoms can worsen. Additionally, the intestines produce hormones like GLP-1 that regulate insulin and appetite; when dysregulated, this can lead to inflammation and blood sugar imbalances.

By the time your food reaches the large intestine (colon), most of the nutrients have been absorbed and what is left is formed into stool. This is also home to your microbiome, the vast collection of bacteria, viruses, and fungi that live in your gut. These microbes feed off the fiber in your stool and produce important postbiotics called short-chain fatty acids (SCFAs), which strengthen your gut lining and support metabolic function.

But if your gut lining is weak, a condition often called "leaky gut", it can lead to systemic inflammation, food intolerances, and even autoimmune issues. And if your microbiome is out of balance, like we saw with Mona's case, it can lead to an overgrowth of harmful pathogens, causing inflammation and digestive problems (more on this later).

The digestive journey ends with waste elimination, but it relies on a delicate balance of enzymes, hormones, gut bacteria, and nervous system signals. If anything goes off track, symptoms like bloating, discomfort, or irregular bowel movements can arise. For us women, keeping this system running smoothly is especially crucial for overall health.

The Root Cause

When women come to me with digestive issues, my goal is to look at the whole picture to find the root cause. So, let us talk about what I look for when your digestion is off, because there are so many pieces to this puzzle.

First, I consider autoimmune diseases. Women are more likely than men to have an undiagnosed autoimmune disease and GI symptoms may be the first sign. Conditions like Sjögren's syndrome can cause dry mouth, thyroid diseases can cause constipation or diarrhea, or scleroderma, which can slow motility, can cause trouble swallowing or bloating. Celiac disease can cause digestive issues, plus rashes and fatigue. And Crohn's disease or Ulcerative colitis can cause weight loss, bowel changes, and anemia. Autoimmunity, as we discussed in Chapter 6, is often overlooked but can play a huge role in digestive symptoms.

Next, I look at medications. Things like antacids can reduce stomach acid, and lead to malabsorption and bacterial overgrowth in the small intestine. Antibiotics, while sometimes necessary, can wreak havoc on your gut microbiome. NSAIDs, birth control pills, statins, chemotherapy, iron supplements, antidepressants, blood pressure medications and opioids can lead to imbalances, which can cause gas, bloating, and irregular bowel movements.

I also check for infections, like H. pylori, which can cause ulcers and gastritis, or other pathogens like bacteria, candida, and parasites, which might be disrupting your gut. And let us not forget about toxins, whether there are additives and pesticides in food, environmental toxins, or even alcohol, these can negatively affect the health of your liver and gut microbiome.

Your genetics matter too. Your liver helps detoxify toxins that we make in our cells and those we consume. Some people have variations in their detoxification pathways, making it harder for their bodies to process and eliminate toxins, which can lead to inflammation and digestive issues. We may also have nutritional deficiencies that are key co-factors on the detoxification process, motility, and hormone secretion.

Then there is pancreatic function. If your pancreas is not producing enough enzymes, your body cannot properly break down fats, proteins, or carbs, leading to malabsorption and symptoms like bloating or diarrhea.

I also consider leaky gut, where the lining of your intestines becomes permeable, allowing undigested food particles and toxins to enter your bloodstream. This can trigger food intolerances, inflammation, and even autoimmune reactions.

Speaking of food intolerances, I always explore whether certain foods are triggering your symptoms. But it is not just about food, mast cell activation can cause your immune system to overreact to everyday triggers, leading to bloating, cramping, or diarrhea.

Hormones play a big role too. Fluctuations in estrogen and progesterone can directly affect your gut microbiome and motility, which is why so many women notice digestive changes during their menstrual cycle, pregnancy, or menopause.

And of course, I cannot ignore stress. Chronic stress impacts the Vagus nerve, which controls digestion. When your Vagus nerve is not functioning well, it can slow motility, reduce stomach acid production, and even contribute to acid reflux.

The truth is, digestion is a complex process, and there is rarely just one thing causing your symptoms. While medications, infections, hormones, and stress all influence digestive health, one master system connects them all: your gut microbiome. Imagine a lush, thriving rainforest, home to trillions of microorganisms that influence every cell in your body.

Now, let us uncover how these mighty microbes do more than improve digestion; they hold the key to your entire well-being.

The Importance of the Gut Microbiome

Your gut microbiome, the trillions of bacteria, viruses, and fungi in your digestive tract, does more than digest food. It influences your brain, heart, hormones, immune system, skin, weight, and mood. When balanced, it keeps your body running smoothly. When out of sync, it can disrupt everything. Keeping your microbiome healthy is key to supporting your whole body. Let us explore how this hidden powerhouse connects to every part of you.

Gut Microbiome and Nutrient Absorption

Your gut microbiome helps break down complex carbohydrates, proteins, and fats that your body cannot digest on its own. It also produces essential nutrients like vitamin K, B vitamins, and short-chain fatty acids (SCFAs), which nourish the cells lining your intestines and support overall gut health. Without a balanced microbiome, you may struggle to absorb key nutrients, leading to deficiencies and related health issues.

Gut Microbiome and Brain Health

Did you know your gut is often called the "second brain"? That is because it has its own network of neurons and produces neurotransmitters with the help of your gut microbiome, like serotonin, dopamine, and GABA. In fact, about 90% of serotonin, the "feel-good" hormone, and 50% of dopamine, the reward hormone, is made in your gut with the help of microbes.

When your microbiome is out of balance, it can disrupt production of feel-good hormones, contributing to mood disorders like anxiety and depression. And the opposite is true as well. Stress can disrupt the microbiome, leading to inflammation and immune dysfunction. This is why improving the gut-brain health often leads to better mental clarity and emotional resilience.

Gut Microbiome and Heart Health

Your gut microbiome even plays a role in your heart health. Certain gut bacteria help regulate cholesterol levels and produce compounds like trimethylamine N-oxide (TMAO), which can increase your risk for heart disease risk. An imbalance in these bacteria may contribute to inflammation, plaque in your arteries, high blood pressure, and other heart-related issues.

Gut Microbiome and Hormone Balance

Your microbiome also helps regulate hormones by influencing the metabolism of estrogen, thyroid hormones, and cortisol. For example, an imbalance in gut bacteria can lead to estrogen dominance, a condition linked to endometriosis, fibroids, and even breast cancer. This is especially relevant for us women, as hormonal fluctuations throughout life—whether during menstruation, pregnancy, or menopause—can directly impact gut health. And vice versa, as hormonal changes can also alter the microbiome, affecting mood and digestion.

Gut Microbiome and Immune Function

About 70% of your immune system resides in your gut.[63] Your microbiome helps train your immune cells to distinguish between harmful invaders and harmless substances. A healthy microbiome promotes a balanced immune response, while dysbiosis (an imbalance in gut bacteria) can lead to chronic inflammation, autoimmune conditions, and increased susceptibility to infections.

Gut Microbiome and Skin Health

Ever heard of the gut-skin axis? It is the connection between your microbiome and skin conditions like acne, eczema, and psoriasis. An imbalanced gut can lead to systemic inflammation, which often shows up on your skin. This is why addressing gut health is a key step in achieving clear, glowing skin.

Gut Microbiome and Weight Management

Your microbiome also influences how your body stores fat, regulates blood sugar, and responds to hunger hormones like leptin and ghrelin. An imbalance in gut bacteria can contribute to weight gain, insulin resistance, and metabolic disorders.

This intricate web of connections underscores why gut health is foundational to overall well-being. When your microbiome is out of balance, it can set off a cascade of issues throughout your body. Conversely, restoring balance to your gut can have far-reaching benefits, from improved digestion to better mental health and beyond.

Thankfully, your gut and your microbiome are resilient. There are practical steps you can take to bring your gut and your whole body back into balance.

How To Fix Your Gut

Ladies, your body has a way of telling you when something is not right. Bloating, weight loss, blood in the stool, abdominal pain, irregular bowel movements, or persistent symptoms like heartburn or fatigue are not just "normal" things to brush off. They are signals from your body that something needs attention.

Before diving into any gut-healing strategies, it is crucial to partner with your doctor to rule out serious health issues. Conditions like celiac disease, inflammatory bowel disease (IBD), infections, or even certain cancers can mimic common digestive complaints. A gastrointestinal specialist may be needed to run tests, provide a diagnosis, and ensure you are on the right path.

Once all life-threatening issues have been ruled out and you are ready to focus on restoring your gut health, the 5 R's framework can be a wonderful roadmap to guide you. Think of it as a step-by-step plan to help your digestive system heal, thrive, and feel its best. Let us break it down together!

1. REMOVE: Clear Out the Bad Stuff

The first step is to remove anything irritating or damaging your gut. This includes not only foods but also environmental toxins, infections, and other stressors. Here's how to tackle this step:

Inflammatory Foods

Certain foods can trigger inflammation in the gut, leading to bloating, discomfort, and other digestive issues. Common culprits include:

- **Gluten**: Found in wheat, barley, and rye, gluten can be particularly problematic for those with sensitivities or celiac disease.
- **Dairy**: Lactose or casein in dairy products can cause issues for some people.
- **Sugar**: Excess sugar feeds harmful bacteria and yeast in the gut, disrupting the balance of your microbiome.
- **Processed foods**: These are often loaded with chemicals, preservatives, artificial dyes, and other additives that can irritate the gut lining.
- **Pesticides and herbicides**: Non-organic produce may contain residues that disrupt gut health. Opt for organic when possible.

To identify which foods are problematic for you, consider working with a healthcare provider to test for food allergies or sensitivities. An elimination diet, where you temporarily remove common trigger foods and then reintroduce them one by one, can also be a helpful tool.

Toxins and Heavy Metals

Your gut can also be affected by environmental toxins and heavy metals, which may come from contaminated water, air, or food. These can disrupt the gut lining and harm beneficial bacteria. Consider testing for heavy metals (like lead, mercury, or arsenic) and working with a professional to safely restore health.

Medications

Certain medications, such as antibiotics, NSAIDs (like ibuprofen), and proton pump inhibitors (PPIs), can interfere with digestion and damage the gut lining. If you are taking these medications regularly, talk to your doctor about alternatives or ways to support your gut while using them.

Infections

Infections in the gut can cause ongoing issues. These may include:
- **Bacterial infections**: Like *H. pylori*, which is linked to stomach ulcers and inflammation. Small Intestinal Bacterial Overgrowth and dysbiosis caused by pathogenic bacteria can lead to GI issues.
- **Parasites**: These can disrupt digestion and nutrient absorption.
- **Yeast overgrowth**: An overgrowth of *Candida* or other yeasts can lead to bloating, fatigue, and cravings for sugar.
- **Mold exposure**: Mold toxins (mycotoxins) can damage the gut lining and weaken the immune system.

If you suspect an infection, testing and treatment with a healthcare provider are essential.

Stressors

Chronic stress, poor sleep, and an overloaded schedule can also harm your gut. Stress hormones like cortisol can disrupt digestion and weaken the gut lining. Prioritizing stress management is a key part of this step.

2. REPLACE: Add Back What's Missing

Once you have cleared out the harmful stuff, it is time to replenish what your gut might be lacking. This step is all about supporting your body's natural digestive processes. Here is what to focus on:

Fiber

Fiber is essential for healthy digestion and gut motility. Aim for at least 30 grams of fiber per day from whole foods like vegetables, fruits, legumes, nuts, seeds, and whole grains. Fiber helps feed your gut bacteria, promotes regular bowel movements, and supports a healthy gut lining.

Digestive Support

- **Digestive enzymes**: These enzymes improve nutrient absorption, especially for those with low pancreatic elastase levels.
- **Bile salts**: These are essential for digesting fats, if you have had your gallbladder removed or have sluggish gallbladder function.
- **Stomach acid**: Low stomach acid can lead to bloating and indigestion often seen in the elderly. Supplements under physician guidance may help.

Micronutrients

Certain micronutrient deficiencies can affect digestion or gut motility. Replenishing these can make a big difference:

- **Magnesium**: Supports muscle relaxation and bowel regularity. Found in leafy greens, nuts, seeds, and dark chocolate.
- **Zinc**: Essential for gut repair and immune function. Found in shellfish, seeds, and legumes.
- **B vitamins**: Important for energy production and gut health. Found in whole grains, eggs, and leafy greens.

If you suspect malabsorption (common in conditions like leaky gut or celiac disease), testing for nutrient deficiencies (like iron, vitamin D, or B12) can help guide supplementation.

3. REINOCULATE: Restore the Good Bacteria

Your gut is home to trillions of bacteria and keeping them balanced is key to good digestion. Here's how to rebuild a healthy gut microbiome:

Probiotic Foods

These are foods that contain live, beneficial bacteria. Include a variety of fermented foods in your diet, such as:

- **Yogurt and kefir:** Contains probiotics like *Lactobacillus* and *Bifidobacterium* species.
- **Sauerkraut and kimchi**: Fermented vegetables packed with probiotics.
- **Tempeh and natto**: Fermented soy products that are great plant-based options.
- **Kombucha**: A fizzy, fermented tea drink.

- **Fermented apple cider vinegar** (ACV): Contains beneficial bacteria and enzymes.
- **Sourdough bread**: Made through natural fermentation, which can be easier to digest.

Prebiotic Foods

Prebiotics are fibers that feed the good bacteria in your gut. Include foods like:

- **Resistant starches**: These act as prebiotics and are found in cooked and cooled potatoes, green bananas, and legumes.
- **Garlic and onions**: Rich in inulin, a type of prebiotic fiber.
- **Asparagus and leeks**: Also, great sources of prebiotics.

Postbiotics

Postbiotics are the beneficial byproducts produced when your gut bacteria break down prebiotics. These include short-chain fatty acids (SCFAs), which support gut health and reduce inflammation.

To boost SCFAs:
Add MCT oil, coconut oil, butter, or ghee to your diet. These healthy fats can support gut healing and energy production.

4. REPAIR: Heal the Gut Lining

If your gut lining is damaged (a condition sometimes called "leaky gut"), it needs time and nutrients to heal. To repair the gut lining, consider:

- **Glutamine**: An amino acid that helps rebuild the intestinal lining.
- **Zinc**: Supports gut repair and immune function.

- **Omega-3 fatty acids**: Found in fish oil, flaxseeds, and walnuts, these reduce inflammation and promote healing.
- **Vitamin A**: Essential for maintaining the integrity of the gut lining. Found in liver, sweet potatoes, and carrots.
- **Vitamin D**: Supports immune function and gut health. Get it from sunlight, fatty fish, or supplements.

Healing the gut lining is like patching up a leaky pipe, it helps prevent toxins and undigested food particles from escaping into your bloodstream, which can cause inflammation and other issues.

5. REBALANCE: Support Your Gut with a Healthy Lifestyle

Finally, it is time to look at the bigger picture. Your gut health is deeply connected to your overall lifestyle. To keep your gut happy and healthy:

- **Manage stress**: Practice relaxation techniques like deep breathing, meditation, or yoga. Consider using the Nerva app, a gut-directed hypnotherapy program designed to reduce stress and improve gut symptoms.
- **Prioritize sleep**: Aim for 7-9 hours of quality sleep each night. Your gut repairs itself while you sleep!
- **Move your body**: Regular exercise helps keep your digestive system running smoothly.

By rebalancing your lifestyle, you create an environment where your gut can thrive long-term.

Putting It All Together

The 5 R's—Remove, Replace, Reinoculate, Repair, and Rebalance—are a simple yet powerful way to restore your gut health. Remember, healing takes time, so be patient with yourself. Start with small, manageable changes, and celebrate each step forward. Your gut is the foundation of your overall health, and by taking care of it, you are investing in a healthier, happier you.

If you are unsure where to start or have persistent symptoms, always reach out to your healthcare provider first.

In addition to dietary and lifestyle changes, certain supplements can support your gut as it heals.

Suggested Supplements for Digestive Health

Digestive supplements can be a valuable part of your wellness plan when combined with a gut-friendly diet and lifestyle. Whether you are working to ease occasional bloating, support gut healing, or address specific conditions like IBS or SIBO, these evidence-based options may provide targeted relief. As always, consult your healthcare provider before starting new supplements, especially if you have chronic digestive issues, take medications, or are managing autoimmune conditions. See Appendix B for a list of these recommended supplements for digestive health.

Final Thoughts

Digestive health is about so much more than what you eat. It is about how your body processes food, how your mind influences your gut, and how your lifestyle supports or undermines your well-being. For us women, the interplay of hormones, stress, and biology makes this even more complex. But as Mona's story shows, with the right approach, it is possible to unravel even the most stubborn digestive issues and reclaim your health.

The key is to look beyond the symptoms and address the root causes. By understanding the unique ways your body works and taking a holistic, personalized approach, you can create a path to healing that honors your whole self—mind, body, and spirit.

Questions To Discuss With Your Doctor:

These questions are designed to help you have a more informed, collaborative conversation with your healthcare provider, so you can get to the root of what is going on and build a plan that supports your mental, emotional, and physical well-being.

1. Could my digestive symptoms (bloating, gas, constipation, diarrhea) be linked to an underlying condition?

Consider: Testing for conditions like small intestinal bacterial overgrowth (SIBO), irritable bowel syndrome (IBS), inflammatory bowel disease (IBD), or celiac disease.

2. Can I get a comprehensive stool analysis to assess my gut health?

Request: Testing for gut microbiome diversity, dysbiosis, leaky gut markers, parasites, yeast overgrowth, and digestive enzyme function.

3. Could food sensitivities or allergies be contributing to my symptoms?

Discuss: Food sensitivity testing or an elimination diet to identify triggers like gluten, dairy, or other allergens.

4. Could my gut health be impacting other areas of my health, like my immune system or mental health?

Consider: The gut-brain connection and how gut imbalances might contribute to mood disorders, fatigue, or autoimmune conditions.

5. Could nutrient deficiencies or malabsorption be playing a role in my symptoms?

Request: Micronutrient testing or organic acid testing to assess levels of key nutrients like B vitamins, magnesium, or zinc.

6. Could chronic stress or adrenal dysfunction be affecting my digestion?

Discuss: Timed salivary cortisol testing to evaluate adrenal function and the impact of stress on gut health.

7. Are there supplements or natural therapies that could support my digestive health?

Consider: Probiotics, digestive enzymes, L-glutamine, or herbal remedies like slippery elm or aloe vera.

8. What dietary changes do you recommend to improve my gut health?

Discuss: Anti-inflammatory diets, low-FODMAP diets, or specific nutrients to support gut healing and microbiome balance.

9. Could my medications (e.g., antibiotics, PPIs) be impacting my gut health?

Consider: How long-term use of medications might disrupt gut flora and explore alternatives or supportive therapies.

10. Can we evaluate my sleep and stress levels, as they impact gut health?

Discuss: Sleep hygiene practices and stress management techniques like meditation, yoga, or deep breathing.

11. Can you refer me to specialists who can help me further?

Consider: A nutritionist for personalized dietary guidance, a gastroenterologist for advanced care, or an integrative medicine practitioner for a comprehensive approach.

12. Can we partner together to create a preventative health plan for my digestive health?

Work with your doctor to develop a personalized plan that addresses your unique needs, symptoms, and goals.

For a complete companion resource, including all "Questions to Discuss with Your Doctor," Supplement Lists, and Guides, scan the QR code.

Chapter 8

Musculoskeletal Health

"The body achieves what the mind believes."

—**Serena Williams**

Meet Mary, a vibrant 65-year-old woman who recently moved to Arizona after retiring from a high-powered executive career. Mary has always been tall, thin, and lean, traits she has carried throughout her life. But ten years ago, she was diagnosed with osteoporosis, a condition marked by thinning bones, and was prescribed medication to slow bone loss. Her family history didn't help, both her mother and sister had osteoporosis as well.

Mary has always been dedicated to her cardio routine and a vegetarian diet, but now, in retirement, she was ready to focus on her health in a way her demanding career never allowed. She was determined to take control of her well-being, and that is what brought her to me, to establish care with a new doctor and start this next chapter of her life on the right foot.

Mary grew up in a middle-class family, but her childhood was not easy. Her father struggled with alcoholism and passed away from esophageal cancer. Both of her parents were smokers, and Mary was exposed to secondhand smoke throughout her formative years.

Despite these challenges, Mary emerged with remarkable resilience and determination.

On examination, Mary was thin, with a low BMI of 17. Her body composition analysis showed lower muscle mass than desired; a condition called sarcopenia. I explained to her that this increases her risk for muscle weakness and bone fractures. Her labs revealed low levels of Vitamin D3, Vitamin B12, and omega-3 fats, along with elevated bone turnover markers. Her repeat bone density scan showed worsening osteoporosis.

Mary's story is a powerful reminder of how our biology, lifestyle, and environment intersect to shape our health. But it is also a story of hope, because as we explore musculoskeletal health together throughout this chapter, you will discover how the right knowledge and tools can help you take control of your health and thrive, no matter your age or circumstances.

The Mitochondrial Connection: Your Cellular Superpower

Mary's journey led me to reflect on the incredible resilience of women. Growing up with immigrant parents, I always marveled at my mom. She was a force of nature, juggling four kids, cooking, cleaning, managing grocery runs, paying bills, and working alongside my dad in his medical office. Somehow, she did not just survive the chaos—she thrived. She handled stress with grace, and I often wondered if she had some kind of superpower.

Years later, I found myself stepping into her shoes, balancing long hours as a physician, managing a household, and being a wife and mother. I pushed myself to the brink, telling myself I had to keep going no matter what. But it made me wonder: What makes us, as women, capable of handling so much? What allows us to adapt to the physical demands of life and keep moving forward, even when we feel like we have hit a wall?

The secret lies, in part, in our mitochondria, the tiny powerhouses inside our cells that produce the energy fueling nearly every function in our bodies. Here's something you may not know, we inherit our mitochondria directly from our mothers, who inherited them from their mothers, and so on. Unlike nuclear DNA, which comes from both parents, mitochondrial DNA is passed down almost exclusively through the maternal line. It is like a biological heirloom, a gift of energy from the women who came before us.

Most studies show that women have a higher mitochondrial content overall, with greater mitochondrial volume density in tissues like skeletal muscle.[64] This difference is not just a scientific curiosity, it has real-world implications for how we move, metabolize energy, and even how long we live.

When our mitochondrial function declines, two silent conditions often emerge: osteoporosis (weakening bones) and sarcopenia (muscle loss). Let us examine how these processes develop at the cellular level, and why your mitochondria are central to both.

Understanding Osteoporosis and Sarcopenia

During Mary's visit, I explained to her that bone and muscle loss are not just related to aging, they are metabolic diseases caused by a combination of factors. Think of it like a tornado: genetics, age, lifestyle, hormones, and even the health of your mitochondria all play a role.

Your mitochondria act as master regulators for bone health, balancing the work of bone-building osteoblasts and bone-resorbing osteoclasts. Bone breakdown can start to outpace bone formation when mitochondria are not working well due to aging, chronic inflammation (caused by things like stress, poor sleep, or a diet high in sugar), oxidative stress (like the damage caused by too many processed foods or that extra glass of wine at happy hour), or poor nutrition (Standard American Diet). Over time, this leads to thinner, more fragile bones that are prone to fractures.

Similarly, in muscles, sarcopenia (muscle loss) happens when muscle breakdown outpaces rebuilding, often due to aging, hormonal changes like menopause, inactivity, poor nutrition, and mitochondrial dysfunction. When mitochondria are not working well, they cannot produce enough energy to keep muscles strong, leading to weakness and wasting. As you age, you also lose muscle fibers, especially the ones needed for strength, and fat can start to infiltrate muscle tissue, making it even weaker.

Risk factors like a sedentary lifestyle, low protein intake, chronic inflammation, smoking, and excessive alcohol can speed up this process. Over time, this can lead to weaker muscles, increased fall risk, slower recovery, and disrupted metabolism.

Let us examine the key players affecting your mitochondrial health and in turn bone and muscle health.

Risk Factors That Affect Mitochondrial Health in Bone and Muscle

Let us break it down so you can understand what might be harming your mitochondria and, in turn, your bones and muscles.

1. Genetics: The Starting Point

If your mother, grandmother, or other close relatives had osteoporosis, weak bones, or muscle loss, you might be at a higher risk. While you cannot change your genes, you can influence how they play out by addressing other factors.

Race also plays a role. Women of Caucasian and Asian descent tend to have a higher risk of osteoporosis compared to African

American or Hispanic women. However, no matter your background, mitochondrial health is something every woman should prioritize.

2. Lifestyle: The Daily Choices That Add Up

Sitting too much and not moving enough can take a toll on your mitochondria, bones, and muscles. And let us talk about diet. If you are eating the "Standard American Diet", foods high in sugar, refined flour, processed foods, and fried items, but low in protein and nutrient-dense whole foods, your mitochondria are not getting the support they need to function well. It is like trying to run a car on low-quality fuel.

Alcohol is another sneaky factor. Drinking more than one glass a day can interfere with your body's ability to absorb key nutrients like calcium and vitamin D, which are essential for bone and muscle health. Over time, excessive alcohol use can weaken your mitochondria, bones, and muscles.

3. Menopause: The Hormonal Shift

The drop in estrogen that comes with menopause does not just affect your bones, it can also impact your mitochondria. Estrogen helps protect your bones and muscles, and when levels drop, your mitochondria may struggle to produce enough energy to keep them strong. This hormonal shift can accelerate bone and muscle loss, making it harder to maintain strength and density.

4. Nutrient Deficiencies: The Silent Saboteurs

Deficiencies in key nutrients like vitamin D, K2, calcium, and magnesium can weaken your mitochondria, bones, and muscles. Vitamin D helps your body absorb calcium, which is the building block of your bones. Vitamin K2 moves the calcium into the bones, while magnesium supports muscle function. If you are not getting enough of these nutrients, your mitochondria cannot do their job properly, and your bones and muscles pay the price.

5. Toxins: The Hidden Culprit

Cigarette smoke, whether firsthand or secondhand, damages your mitochondria, creating inflammation and oxidative stress that weakens bones and muscles. Air pollution, heavy metals (like lead and cadmium), and endocrine-disrupting chemicals in plastics, pesticides, and personal care products can also harm your bone and muscle health. Even household cleaners and cosmetics can contribute. Reducing exposure by choosing natural products, avoiding plastics, and eating organic can help protect your mitochondria and keep your bones and muscles stronger.

Now that we have covered the risk factors, let us explore the steps you can take to build stronger bones and muscles, starting with nutrition.

Bone Health Prescription

Taking care of your bones is more than just taking medication, it is about nourishing your cells, protecting your mitochondria, staying active, and making smart lifestyle choices. Here is a clear, organized plan to help you build stronger bones and prevent further bone loss:

Foods to Include Daily

- **Calcium**: Collard greens, kale, soybeans, Bok choy, figs, broccoli, oranges, sardines, salmon, Greek yogurt
- **Vitamin D3**: Salmon, herring, sardines, eggs, mushrooms, sunlight
- **Magnesium**: Dark chocolate, avocados, nuts, legumes, tofu, seeds

- **Potassium**: Bananas, oranges, potatoes, sweet potatoes, spinach, mushrooms
- **Silicon**: Oats, cucumbers, rice, flaxseeds, avocados
- **Vitamin K** (M7): Natto, cheese, egg yolks, dark chicken meat
- **Boron**: Apricots, peanut butter, Brazil nuts, prunes, lentils
- **Vitamin C**: Broccoli, Brussels sprouts, spinach, sweet potatoes, tomatoes
- **Copper**: Oysters, nuts, seeds, shiitake mushrooms, dark chocolate
- **Zinc**: Oysters, crab, mussels, pine nuts, chickpeas, quinoa
- **Manganese**: Mussels, wheat germ, tofu, sweet potatoes, spinach

Stopping Bone Loss

- **Avoid Harmful Habits**: Steer clear of carbonated sodas, coffee, and alcohol, as they can weaken bones. Never smoke cigarettes.
- **Ditch the Standard American Diet**: Avoid dairy, sugar, flour, meat, processed foods, artificial colors, dyes, and preservatives.
- **Check for Underlying Issues**: Get tested for thyroid, parathyroid, and kidney problems, as these can impact bone health.
- **Be Cautious with Medications**: Avoid long-term use of antacids, PPIs, and steroids, as they can harm bones.

Building Strong Bones

- **Exercise Smart**: Add resistance training 3 days a week to build muscle and bone strength. Keep up cardio 2 days a week. Add a daily walking program and try a vibration plate or rebounder for extra bone support. Work with a physical therapist who specializes in osteoporosis.

- **Optimize Vitamin D3**: Maximize your Vitamin D3 intake and check your levels every 6 months, aiming for a level of 50-60.
- **Alkalize Your Diet**: Focus on dark leafy greens, fruits, vegetables, and plant-based meals.

Now that you have a plan to support bone health, let us explore why weight loss feels harder for women and how your metabolism, mitochondria, and hormones all play a role.

Metabolic Rate: Why Weight Loss Feels Harder for Women

Ever feel like the men in your life can shed weight almost effortlessly, while your body seems to hold onto every last bit of stubborn fat? You are not imagining it, it is biology. As women, our bodies are built to be efficient, meaning we are experts at conserving and using energy over time, rather than burning through it quickly like men do.

It reminds me of how growing up, my mom never threw anything away. She would reuse margarine tubs for leftovers, wash out Ziploc bags, and find a second life for just about everything. Well, in a similar way, our bodies are designed to hold onto energy stores, a survival mechanism that likely evolved to support things like pregnancy and breastfeeding. So, while it might feel frustrating at times, it is also a reminder of how incredible and resilient our bodies are.

We also burn calories differently than men because of our mitochondria. As women, we have a greater number and density of mitochondria in our muscles compared to men, which influences how we burn energy and manage weight. Our muscle fibers are primarily red and slow twitch, packed with mitochondria, making them more efficient at burning calories slowly and excelling in endurance activities. In contrast, men tend to have more white fast-twitch muscle fibers, which allow them to burn calories more quickly. This biological difference highlights how our bodies are uniquely adapted for different energy needs and functions.

This efficiency is a double-edged sword. While it helps us excel in endurance activities, it can make weight loss feel like an uphill battle, especially as we age. Add to this the hormonal changes that come with menopause, which can slow metabolism even further, and it is no wonder those extra pounds feel so stubborn. Meanwhile, men seem to drop weight with less effort, thanks to their faster metabolic rate, more fast-twitch muscle fibers, and higher muscle mass.

The good news? You are not stuck with this metabolic setup. Women's bodies are incredibly adaptable, and we can work with our biology to boost our metabolic rate, build muscle, and lose fat. Here is how:

Strategies to Lose Fat: Science-Backed Steps You Can Start Today

1. Strength Training: Build Muscle to Boost Metabolism

Muscle burns more calories at rest than fat, so building lean muscle is key to revving up your metabolism. Studies show that women who engage in regular strength training lose more fat and maintain muscle mass better than those who focus solely on cardio.

- **What to do:** Aim for 2-3 strength training sessions per week, focusing on compound movements like squats, deadlifts, lunges, and push-ups.

> **Pro tip:** Lift heavy enough that the last 2-3 reps of each set feel challenging. Progressive overload (gradually increasing weight or resistance) is essential for building muscle.

2. High-Intensity Interval Training (HIIT): Burn Fat in Less Time

HIIT is a game-changer for women because it combines the fat-burning benefits of cardio with the metabolic boost of strength training. Research shows that HIIT can increase fat loss while preserving muscle mass, making it ideal for women's bodies.[65]

- **What to do:** Try a 20-30 minute HIIT workout 2-3 times per week. For example, alternate 30 seconds of sprinting, jumping jacks, or burpees with 1 minute of walking or rest.

> **Pro tip:** Add resistance to your HIIT workouts (like using dumbbells or kettlebells) to further boost calorie burn and muscle engagement. Aim for HIIT in the first half of your menstrual cycle (if it applies). Avoid HIIT during times of mental and physical stress.

3. Prioritize Protein: Fuel Muscle Growth and Curb Cravings

Protein is essential for building and repairing muscle, and it also helps keep you full longer. Studies show that a high-protein diet can boost metabolism, reduce appetite, and support fat loss, especially in women.

⊃ **What to do:** Aim for 20-30 grams of protein per meal. Include lean sources like chicken, fish, eggs, Greek yogurt, tofu, or legumes.

Pro tip: Have a protein-rich snack (like a hard-boiled egg or a protein shake) within 30 minutes after your workout to support muscle recovery and growth.

4. Incorporate NEAT: Move More Throughout the Day

Non-Exercise Activity Thermogenesis (NEAT), the calories you burn through daily activities like walking, cleaning, or fidgeting, can make a big difference in weight loss. Women's bodies are naturally efficient at endurance, so take advantage of this by staying active throughout the day.

⊃ **What to do:** Aim for 8,000-10,000 steps per day. Take the stairs, park farther away, or do a 10-minute walk after meals.

Pro tip: Use a fitness tracker to monitor your daily activity and set small, achievable goals.

5. Manage Stress and Sleep: Support Hormonal Balance

Chronic stress and poor sleep can disrupt hormones like cortisol and insulin, making it harder to lose fat. Add in restorative exercises instead of high intensity workouts. Studies show that women who prioritize sleep and stress management are more successful at losing weight and keeping it off.

- **What to do**: Aim for 7-9 hours of quality sleep per night. Practice stress-reducing activities like yoga, meditation, or deep breathing exercises.

Pro tip: Create a bedtime routine to improve sleep quality, such as avoiding screens an hour before bed and keeping your bedroom cool and dark.

Now that we have explored how to optimize our metabolism and fat loss, let us talk about another biological superpower our mitochondria give us as women: longevity.

Lifespan: The Mitochondrial Longevity Advantage

Did you know that women, on average, live longer than men? While genetics, lifestyle, and healthcare access all play a role, our mitochondria might be one of the hidden reasons. Women's higher mitochondrial content and efficiency not only help us sustain energy but also protect our cells from damage over time, contributing to our longer lifespan.

Mitochondria are like the batteries of our cells. When they are functioning well, they reduce oxidative stress and inflammation, two major drivers of aging. Women's bodies are also better at repairing mitochondrial damage, which may explain why we tend to outlive men. But this advantage is not a guarantee. Chronic stress, poor nutrition, and environmental toxins can still take a toll on our mitochondria, speeding up aging and increasing the risk of age-related diseases.

The good news? You can take steps today to support your mitochondria and unlock your longevity potential. Here is how:

Practical Solutions to Boost Mitochondrial Health

Your mitochondria are the powerhouses of your cells, and keeping them healthy is key to maintaining energy, vitality, and longevity. Here are science-backed strategies to support your mitochondrial health and lifespan:

1. Eat the Rainbow: Fuel Your Mitochondria with Antioxidants

Antioxidants help neutralize free radicals, which can damage mitochondria and accelerate aging. Colorful fruits and vegetables are packed with these protective compounds.

- **What to do:** Aim to fill half your plate with a variety of colorful produce at every meal. Think berries, leafy greens, bell peppers, carrots, and sweet potatoes.

> **Pro tip:** Add herbs and spices like turmeric, ginger, and cinnamon to your meals, they are rich in antioxidants and anti-inflammatory compounds.

2. Move Daily: Exercise to Strengthen Mitochondria

Regular physical activity has been shown to boost mitochondrial function and even increase the number of mitochondria in your cells. Both aerobic exercise and strength training are beneficial.

- **What to do:** Aim for at least 150 minutes of moderate aerobic activity (like brisk walking or cycling) per week, plus 2-3 strength training sessions.

> **Pro tip:** Try interval training (like alternating between walking and jogging) to maximize mitochondrial benefits in less time.

3. Prioritize Sleep: Repair and Recharge Your Cells

Sleep is when your body repairs cellular damage, including damage to mitochondria. Poor sleep can increase oxidative stress and impair mitochondrial function.

- **What to do:** Aim for 7-9 hours of quality sleep each night. Create a calming bedtime routine by avoiding screens, dimming lights, and practicing relaxation techniques.

> **Pro tip:** Keep your bedroom cool (around 65°F or 18°C) and dark to promote deeper sleep.

4. Manage Stress: Protect Your Mitochondria from Wear and Tear

Chronic stress increases inflammation and oxidative stress, both of which harm mitochondria. Stress management techniques can help protect your cells and support longevity.

- **What to do:** Incorporate daily stress-reducing practices like yoga, meditation, deep breathing, or even a 10-minute walk in nature.

Pro tip: Try mindfulness apps or guided meditation if you are new to stress management techniques.

5. Avoid Toxins: Reduce Mitochondrial Damage

Environmental toxins like cigarette smoke, air pollution, and chemicals in household products can damage mitochondria and accelerate aging.

- **What to do:** Avoid smoking and secondhand smoke, use natural cleaning products, and choose organic foods when possible, to reduce exposure to pesticides.

Pro tip: Invest in an air purifier for your home to reduce indoor air pollution.

6. Stay Hydrated: Support Cellular Function

Water is essential for mitochondrial function and overall cellular health. Dehydration can impair energy production and increase oxidative stress.

- **What to do:** Aim to drink at least 8 cups (64 ounces) of water daily, more if you are active or live in a hot climate.

Pro tip: Start your day with a glass of water and carry a reusable water bottle to stay hydrated throughout the day.

7. Intermittent Fasting: Boost Mitochondrial Efficiency

Intermittent fasting has been shown to improve mitochondrial function by promoting cellular repair processes like autophagy, where cells remove damaged components and recycle them.

- **What to do:** Try a 12–16 hour fasting window each day (e.g., eating between 8 a.m. and 6 p.m.). Start with shorter fasts and gradually increase the duration.

Pro tip: Stay hydrated with water, herbal tea, or black coffee during your fasting window. Avoid fasting during times of mental or physical stress.

8. Red Light Therapy: Energize Your Mitochondria

Red light therapy uses low-wavelength red light to penetrate the skin and stimulate mitochondrial energy production. Studies suggest it can improve cellular repair and reduce inflammation.

- ⮕ **What to do:** Use a red-light therapy device for 10-20 minutes per session, 3-5 times per week. Focus on areas of the body with thin skin, like the face, neck, or hands.

> **Pro tip:** Look for FDA-cleared devices like Joovv and follow the manufacturer's guidelines for safe use.

9. Sauna Therapy: Heat for Cellular Health

Regular sauna use has been linked to improved mitochondrial function, reduced inflammation, and increased longevity. The heat stress from saunas triggers a protective response in cells, boosting mitochondrial efficiency.

- ⮕ **What to do:** Aim for 2-3 sauna sessions per week, lasting 15-20 minutes each. Stay hydrated and cool down gradually afterward.

> **Pro tip:** If you do not have access to a sauna, try a warm bath with Epsom salts for similar benefits. Women benefit more from heat therapy than cold.

10. Cold Therapy: Shock Your Mitochondria into Action

Cold exposure, like cold showers or ice baths, can stimulate mitochondrial biogenesis, the creation of new mitochondria. It also reduces inflammation and improves energy metabolism.

- **What to do:** Start with 30–60 seconds of cold water at the end of your shower and gradually increase the duration. Alternatively, try an ice bath for 2–5 minutes.

> **Pro tip:** Breathe deeply and stay calm during cold exposure to help your body adapt. For women, benefits begin at temperatures as mild as 50°F (10°C), no extreme cold needed.

As we continue exploring the strengths rooted in our mitochondrial biology, let us talk about one of the most powerful gifts women possess, our natural endurance.

Endurance Is Our Superpower

Ever notice how the hour-long aerobics, dance, or Zumba classes that require long endurance are packed with women, while men often dominate the weight room? It is not just a cultural preference, it is biology. Women are built for endurance and fatigue resistance because we tend to have a higher proportion of slow-twitch Type I muscle fibers. These fibers are rich in mitochondria, allowing us to sustain steady, prolonged effort more efficiently. Studies even show that women's muscles are better at using fat as fuel during endurance activities, helping us conserve energy over time. This mitochondrial efficiency is like having a built-in energy reserve that keeps us going, even when we feel like we have hit our limit.

While men have more fast-twitch Type II fibers, which tire out quickly but produce stronger, faster bursts of power (think sprinting or weightlifting), women's bodies are naturally wired to excel in endurance. This does not mean we can't build strength, speed, or muscle, we absolutely can. It just means we must approach it differently. By incorporating strength training, plyometrics, and targeted nutrition, we can build power and muscle while still leveraging our natural endurance advantage.

How to Build Strength and Power as a Woman

1. Strength Training: Lift Heavy to Build Muscle

Strength training is essential for building muscle and boosting metabolism. While women excel in endurance, lifting weights can help us develop the fast-twitch fibers needed for power and strength.

- ⮕ **What to do:** Aim for 2-3 strength training sessions per week, focusing on compound movements like squats, deadlifts, bench presses, and rows.

> **Pro tip:** Lift heavy enough that the last 2-3 reps of each set feel challenging. Gradually increase the weight or resistance to keep progressing.

2. Plyometrics: Train for Explosive Power

Plyometric exercises, like jump squats, box jumps, and burpees, help develop fast-twitch muscle fibers and improve explosive power.

- **What to do:** Add 1-2 plyometric workouts per week. Start with 3-4 sets of 8-10 reps for exercises like jump squats or box jumps.

> **Pro tip:** Focus on proper form to avoid injury, and land softly to protect your joints.

3. High-Intensity Interval Training (HIIT): Combine Strength and Endurance

HIIT workouts combine the fat-burning benefits of cardio with the muscle-building benefits of strength training. They are a great way to build power while still leveraging your natural endurance.

- **What to do:** Try a 20-30 minute HIIT workout 2-3 times per week. Alternate between 30 seconds of high-intensity exercises (like sprints or kettlebell swings) and 1 minute of rest or low-intensity movement.

> **Pro tip:** Add resistance to your HIIT workouts (like dumbbells or resistance bands) to further challenge your muscles. Focus on HIIT in the first half of your menstrual cycle (if it applies). Avoid HIIT during times of stress.

4. Targeted Nutrition: Fuel Your Muscles for Growth

To build strength and power, your body needs the right fuel. Protein, in particular, is essential for muscle repair and growth.

- **What to do:** Aim for 20–30 grams of protein per meal. Include lean sources like chicken, fish, eggs, Greek yogurt, tofu, or legumes.

> **Pro tip:** Have a protein-rich snack (like a hard-boiled egg or a protein shake) within 30 minutes after your workout to support muscle recovery.

5. Recovery: Rest and Repair

Building strength and power requires more than just exercise; it also requires proper recovery. Rest allows your muscles to repair and grow stronger.

- **What to do:** Aim for 7–9 hours of quality sleep each night. Incorporate active recovery days with light activities like walking, yoga, or stretching.

> **Pro tip:** Use foam rolling or massage therapy to reduce muscle soreness and improve recovery. Plan on more rest and recovery in the second half of your menstrual cycle (if it applies).

The Bottom Line

Women's bodies are naturally wired for endurance, but that does not mean we cannot build strength, speed, and power. By incorporating strength training, plyometrics, HIIT, and targeted nutrition into your routine, you can develop the fast-twitch fibers needed for explosive power while still leveraging your natural endurance advantage. Start today by adding one or two of these strategies to your workouts. Remember, it is not about comparing yourself to men, it is about understanding your body and giving it the tools it needs to thrive. With the right approach, you can build a stronger, more powerful version of yourself while staying true to your biology.

Suggested Supplements for Musculoskeletal Health

Bone, muscle and joint health are best supported through a combination of proper nutrition, regular low-impact exercise, and targeted supplementation. See Appendix B for a list of these recommended supplements for musculoskeletal health.

Final Thoughts

Understanding how our bodies are wired lets us create fitness routines that match our strengths. In this chapter, we have explored how to make the most of your natural endurance while building muscle, boosting metabolism, and supporting bone health. While we may need to approach strength and high-intensity training differently, tailoring them to our hormones and recovery needs, we are just as capable of building power and resilience as men. It is about working with our unique biology, not against it, and celebrating what our bodies are designed to do.

Let us embrace our strength, honor our bodies, and build a future where we thrive, not in spite of our biology, but because of it.

Questions To Discuss With Your Doctor:

These questions are designed to help you have a more informed, collaborative conversation with your healthcare provider, so you can get to the root of what is going on and build a plan that supports your mental, emotional, and physical well-being.

1. Could my symptoms (muscle weakness, joint pain, stiffness, or slow recovery) be linked to an underlying condition?

Consider: Testing for conditions like vitamin D deficiency, osteoporosis, osteoarthritis, rheumatoid arthritis, or autoimmune diseases like lupus or polymyositis.

2. Can I get lab work to assess my nutrient levels and musculoskeletal health?

Request: Testing for vitamin D, calcium, magnesium, potassium, phosphorus, B vitamins, parathyroid hormone (PTH), and inflammatory markers like hs-CRP or IL-6.

3. Could my bone health be impacted by hormonal imbalances?

Discuss: Testing for thyroid function (TSH, free T3, free T4, reverse T3), sex hormones (estrogen, progesterone, testosterone), and cortisol levels.

4. Could chronic inflammation or autoimmune conditions be affecting my muscles, bones, or joints?

Consider: Testing for autoimmune markers like ANA, rheumatoid factor (RF), anti-CCP, or myositis-specific antibodies if muscle weakness or joint pain is present.

5. Could my diet or nutrient absorption be contributing to my symptoms?

Request: Micronutrient testing or organic acid testing to assess levels of key nutrients like calcium, magnesium, vitamin K2, or amino acids.

6. Are there supplements or natural therapies that could support my muscle, bone, and joint health?

Consider: Vitamin D, calcium, magnesium, omega-3 fatty acids, collagen, glucosamine, chondroitin, or anti-inflammatory herbs like turmeric or boswellia.

7. Could my exercise routine or recovery practices be impacting my musculoskeletal health?

Discuss: Overtraining, improper recovery, or the need for tailored exercise plans to support strength, flexibility, and joint mobility.

8. What dietary changes do you recommend to support muscle, bone, and joint health?

Discuss: Anti-inflammatory diets, adequate protein intake, and foods rich in calcium, magnesium, vitamin K2, and antioxidants.

9. Could my medications (e.g., statins, corticosteroids) be affecting my muscles, bones, or joints?

Consider: How medications might contribute to muscle pain, bone loss, or joint stiffness and explore alternatives or supportive therapies.

10. Can we evaluate my sleep and stress levels, as they impact recovery and musculoskeletal health?

Discuss: Sleep hygiene practices and stress management techniques like meditation, yoga, or deep breathing.

11. Can you refer me to specialists who can help me further?

Consider: A nutritionist for personalized dietary guidance, a physical therapist for tailored exercise plans, or a Rheumatologist for a comprehensive approach.

12. Can we partner together to create a preventative health plan for my muscle, bone, and joint health?

Work with your doctor to develop a personalized plan that addresses your unique needs, symptoms, and goals.

For a complete companion resource, including all "Questions to Discuss with Your Doctor," Supplement Lists, and Guides, scan the QR code.

Part 2

Beyond Knowledge: Turn Awareness into Action

Chapter 9

Speak Up: Communicating with Yourself and Your Doctor

"The cost of silence is far greater than the risk of speaking up."

—Brené Brown

Let me tell you about Amy, a 31-year-old new mother whose journey changed the way I think about resilience and self-advocacy. Amy had always been vibrant and active and loved hiking with her husband, traveling with friends, and hitting the gym regularly. Movement was her joy, her escape, her way of life. But one day, while carrying a backpack through the airport on a trip, she felt a sharp, deep ache in her back. By the end of the trip, the pain had become so excruciating that she had to hand her bag to her husband. From that day forward, her life changed. The pain waxed and waned, some days leaving her unable to get out of bed.

Amy sought help from multiple doctors. She saw orthopedists, spine surgeons, rheumatologists and even a neurologist. Each one ran tests, shrugged their shoulders, and told her they couldn't find anything wrong. She was passed from one specialist to another, each visit leaving her feeling more unheard, more unseen, and more alone. Have you ever felt like that? Like you are being shuffled from doctor to doctor without getting answers, without being truly seen?

But here is where Amy's story takes a turn and offers us all a powerful lesson. She became pregnant with her first child, and after giving birth, the pain intensified. Severe lower back pain in her sacroiliac (SI) joints radiated to her upper neck and shoulders, becoming so debilitating that she could barely care for her newborn or walk without wincing in pain. Imagine trying to cradle your baby, only to feel like your body was betraying you with every movement. Through the frustration, a fierce determination was born, a resolve to figure out what was going on.

Instead of giving up, Amy chose to rise. She decided enough was enough and took control of her health. She started keeping a detailed log of her symptoms, tracking when the pain flared up, what made it worse, and what provided even the slightest relief. She created a binder with all her test results, imaging reports, and notes from her appointments. She researched her symptoms, joined online communities of women with similar experiences, and armed herself with knowledge.

And then, finally, we met. Amy was diagnosed with an autoimmune condition called Ankylosing Spondylitis. Amy did not just rely on her diagnosis. She became her own best doctor. She learned to communicate with herself first. She knew the patterns of her pain. She tracked what foods triggered it, which activities worsened it, and how stress and sleep impacted her symptoms. She tracked the effects of her therapies and medications meticulously, so she could communicate clearly with her doctors. She was not afraid to ask about cutting-edge treatments, medications, or therapies.

Amy engaged in physical therapy, targeted exercises, and lifestyle adjustments. Slowly but surely, she began to heal. She worked tirelessly to regain her ability to care for her baby, to move without pain, and to feel like herself again. She connected with support groups for her condition, finding resources and sharing what she had learned along the way.

Amy's story is not just inspiring, it provides a blueprint for others. It is a testament to the power of self-advocacy. It is a reminder that you do not have to suffer in silence or accept dismissive answers. You have the power to take charge of your health, to speak up, and to demand the care you deserve.

She proved that even the most prepared patient can face a medical system slow to listen. Let us examine why this happens and how you can overcome it.

Do Doctors Have a 'God Complex?

So why did Amy's doctors not believe her? As a practicing doctor for over twenty years, I can speak from experience. The medical profession often attracts individuals who are perfectionists, driven by a desire to solve problems and heal others. We pride ourselves on knowing the answers, and our training reinforces the idea that we should always have a solution. This mindset, while well-intentioned, can sometimes lead to what is colloquially referred to as a "God complex", a belief that we are infallible or all-knowing. This is not universal, of course, but it is a tendency that can emerge when the pressure to perform meets the fear of failure.

Doctors are trained to rely on evidence, tests, and data. When those tests come back normal, as they often do in complex or poorly understood conditions like Amy's, it can be frustrating. We want to help, but when we cannot find a clear answer, it challenges our sense of competence. This fear of failure, combined with the need to maintain the respect of our peers and patients, can trigger a fight, flight, or freeze response. Some doctors may become defensive or dismissive, others may avoid difficult conversations, and some may simply retreat emotionally, becoming unavailable to their patients. It is human nature. But it is a flaw in the system that can leave patients like Amy feeling abandoned and unheard.

That is why cultivating humility and curiosity in medicine is so essential. Amy's experience highlights a critical gap in modern medicine: the need for humility and collaboration. The best physicians recognize this and are willing to say, "I don't know, but I will work with you to find out." They listen to their patients, value their lived experiences, and see them as partners in the healing process. Amy's journey is a powerful reminder that medicine is not just about diagnosing and treating, it is about connecting, understanding, and advocating together. Her story challenges us to do better, to be better, and to remember that the patient's voice is just as important as the doctor's expertise.

How to Make the Most of Your Doctor's Visit

I have had the privilege of working with patients from all walks of life. Some come into my office prepared with stacks of papers, detailed logs of their symptoms, and a list of thoughtful questions. Others arrive with little to no knowledge of their medical history or even the medications they are taking. I understand that seeing the doctor can be intimidating. There is often an unspoken assumption that your doctor knows more than you, that they hold all the answers. But here's the truth: you know yourself better than any doctor ever could, especially in the limited time of a fifteen-minute office visit.

Let me pull back the curtain for a moment. Your doctor has thousands of patients, a packed schedule, and barely enough time to catch their breath between appointments. With the demands of paperwork, administrative tasks, and staying on schedule, they may not have had the chance to review your chart before walking into the room. This is not an excuse; it is the reality of our healthcare system.

But it is also why you hold the power to make those fifteen minutes count.

So how do you turn a rushed doctor's visit into a productive and empowering conversation?

To help you get the most out of your appointments and to ensure you leave feeling heard, understood, and with a clear plan, I want to share three steps you can start taking today. These steps will help you walk into your next appointment with confidence, clarity, and the tools you need to advocate for your health. Because at the end of the day, your health is your journey, and you deserve to be in the driver's seat.

Step 1: Confidence—Know Yourself

Before you can communicate clearly with your doctor, you must start by tuning into yourself. The first step is about building confidence in understanding your own body. Too often, we go to the doctor feeling disorganized and overwhelmed. We might not even fully process our concerns before we are in the exam room. By the time we finally articulate what is wrong, our time is up, leaving us frustrated and without solutions.

So, how do we change this? It starts with learning to truly listen to your body. Pay attention to the details, what you are feeling, when it happens, and what makes it better or worse. Write it all down if you can. Those notes will be your secret weapon when you are sitting in the exam room, helping you feel confident, prepared, and in control.

The clearer you are about your symptoms, the easier it is for your doctor to understand what's going on. They will be able to pinpoint the most likely diagnosis, order the right tests, or recommend a treatment plan that works for you. Remember, this is your body. You are the one living in it, feeling it, and experiencing it every single day. That makes you the expert. Own that.

1. **Onset**
    - What is the problem?
    - When did the symptom or problem start?
    - Did it begin suddenly or gradually?
    - Was there a specific event or trigger that caused it?
    - Example: *"The pain started two weeks ago after I lifted a heavy box."*

2. **Location**
    - Where exactly is the symptom located?
    - Is it in one spot, or does it move around?
    - Example: *"The pain is in my lower back, on the right side."*

3. **Duration**
    - How long does the symptom last when it occurs?
    - Is it constant, or does it come and go?
    - Example: *"The pain lasts for about an hour and then goes away, but it comes back every day."*

4. **Characteristics**
    - What does the symptom feel like? (e.g., sharp, dull, throbbing, burning, aching)
    - Are there any other sensations associated with it?
    - Example: *"The pain is sharp and stabbing, and sometimes it feels like it's shooting down my leg."*

5. **Aggravating and Alleviating Factors**
    - What makes the symptom worse? (e.g., movement, certain foods, stress)
    - What makes it better? (e.g., rest, medication, heat)
    - Example: *"The pain gets worse when I sit for too long, but it feels better when I lie down."*

6. **Radiation**
    - Does the symptom spread or move to other areas of the body?
    - Example: *"The pain starts in my lower back but radiates down my right leg."*

7. **Timing**
    - When does the symptom occur? (e.g., morning, night, after eating, during exercise)
    - Has it changed over time?
    - Example: *"The pain is worse in the morning when I first wake up."*

8. **Severity**
    - How severe is the symptom on a scale of 1 to 10?
    - Is it interfering with your daily activities?
    - Example: *"The pain is a 7 out of 10, and it's making it hard for me to walk."*

But do not stop there. Dig deeper. Are there other symptoms that happen at the same time? For example, do you also have a fever, nausea, dizziness, or fatigue? These details can be crucial clues for your doctor.

Think back, have you experienced these symptoms before? If so, how were they treated? Did anything help, or did it make things worse? And finally, how is this affecting your life? Are you struggling to sleep, missing work, or finding it hard to keep up with your daily activities?

When you walk into that exam room with answers to these questions, you are not just a patient. You are an active partner in your care. And that is where real change begins.

Why These Questions Matter

Now that you have reflected on your symptoms, it is important to understand how this preparation translates into better care. These questions help your doctor build a complete picture of your symptoms, which are essential for making an accurate diagnosis and creating an effective treatment plan. By preparing answers to these questions ahead of time, you can ensure your visit is productive and focused on your needs.

One of the most critical pieces of advice I can give you is this: be clear on the top one or two things you want to address during your visit. If you bring a laundry list of a million concerns, you are likely to leave without a meaningful plan and you might miss addressing the most important issues entirely.

I remember a patient who came in concerned about a breast lump. Understandably anxious, she first discussed several other health questions and only mentioned the lump as our time was ending. While we addressed it immediately, I realized how easily important issues can get rushed at the end of an appointment. This experience taught me a valuable lesson I now share with all my patients: *Start with what matters most to you.* Your priorities deserve space and attention and sharing them upfront helps ensure we can give them the focus they need.

In preparation, take time the night before your appointment to organize your thoughts. Write down your top concerns and prioritize them. If you have multiple issues, consider scheduling a separate visit to address them fully. This way, you can ensure that the most pressing matters get the attention they deserve.

Remember, with the current state of managed healthcare, your doctor has little control over the amount of time they can spend with you, but your health is invaluable. By coming prepared, focused, and clear on your priorities, you will not only make the most of your appointment but also take a powerful step toward owning your health journey.

Step 2: Research and Understand Your Problem

Once you have gained clarity about your symptoms, the next step is to educate yourself and this is where your curiosity becomes your strength. It is all about doing your homework and trust me, it is worth the effort. Taking the time to understand your symptoms and research your condition can make a world of difference. Remember, you do not have to do this alone. As women, we are naturally tribal; we thrive in communities. Whether it is your friends, family, colleagues, or even trusted online groups, these connections can be invaluable resources.

The women in your life can help in so many ways. They might recommend a great doctor, point you to vetted sources of information, or connect you with support groups where you can share your story and hear from others who have been through something similar. Sometimes, just hearing about someone else's diagnosis or journey can give you the clarity or answers you have been searching for. And do not forget, your journey can also support someone else who is just starting out and could use your guidance. This is how we lift each other up.

That said, not all information is created equal. When researching, make sure you are looking at vetted, evidence-based sources. Avoid falling down the rabbit hole of unverified claims or anecdotal advice. Instead, seek out reliable websites, medical journals, or organizations that specialize in your condition. If you are not sure where to start, I have included a list of trusted resources at the end of this book to guide you.

The more you know, the more prepared you will be to have a productive discussion with your doctor. Knowledge truly is power. When you walk into that exam room armed with solid information, you are no longer just a patient, you are a partner in your care. And that is where real progress begins.

But let me share a cautionary tale. I once had a patient, Maria, who was desperate for answers after months of unexplained fatigue and joint pain. Frustrated by the lack of clarity from her traditional doctors, she turned to a self-proclaimed "wellness expert" she found online. This person convinced Maria she had a rare parasite and sold her thousands of dollars' worth of supplements and unproven tests. Not only did Maria's symptoms not improve, but she also ended up with new digestive issues from the unregulated supplements. By the time she came to me, she was emotionally drained, financially strained, and no closer to a real diagnosis.

Maria's story is a reminder of how important it is to seek out credible, evidence-based information. While it is tempting to look for quick fixes or alternative solutions, unverified advice can lead you down a dangerous path. Stick to trusted sources, and do not hesitate to bring what you have learned to your doctor for discussion.

So, take the time to research. Ask questions. Lean on your community. And remember, you are not just doing this for yourself, you are setting an example for every woman who has ever felt dismissed or unheard. Your journey can inspire and guide others, creating a ripple effect of empowerment and change. Let us change the narrative to one informed conversation at a time.

Step 3: Ask—Communicate Your Needs

Now that you have gained clarity on your symptoms and done your research, it is time to step into the exam room and speak up for yourself with purpose and poise. You are ready to walk into the doctor's office with confidence and a solid understanding of your symptoms. You are prepared to partner with your doctor on the next steps. But how you communicate matters just as much as what you say. Often, patients enter the exam room in fight, flight, or freeze mode. They are stressed, overwhelmed, and may anticipate resistance, which can come off as confrontational. This does not help the situation, as it may make the doctor defensive if you are angry or demanding. Others might become overly agreeable or passive-aggressive, not clearly expressing their concerns, which makes it hard for the doctor to know if their recommendations are truly meeting your needs. And some may sit in silence, "frozen" and disconnected from the conversation, unable to recall what was discussed when asked by family members later.

On the other hand, your doctor might be having a tough day, running behind, juggling multiple tasks, or putting out fires before the day ends. This means you may not have their full, undivided attention. Studies show that after seconds of someone speaking, humans tend to get distracted by their own thoughts, and doctors are no exception. They might catch the beginning of what you say, form their own conclusions, and start thinking about tests or treatments before you have finished explaining.

Whether it is your spouse, co-worker, child, parent, or doctor, communication is the key to a successful relationship. By approaching the conversation with clarity, calmness, and collaboration, you can ensure your voice is heard and your needs are met.

Let me introduce you to the conscious communication model, a simple, effective way to ensure your voice is heard while keeping the conversation collaborative and productive.

1. **First, create safety.** Start by acknowledging your trust in your doctor's expertise and expressing that you are both on the same team. For example, you might say, "I really value your knowledge and experience, and I know we both want to figure this out together." This sets a tone of collaboration, not confrontation.
2. **Next, state the facts** about your problem concisely and clearly. Share what you have noticed about your symptoms, when they started, and how they have been affecting you. Everything you

prepared the night before. For instance, "I've been experiencing sharp lower back pain for the past three weeks, and it's making it hard for me to sleep or pick up my baby."

3. **Then, ask for what you need.** Be specific about what you are looking for, whether it is tests, a referral to a specialist, or a clearer explanation of your symptoms. For example, "I would like to explore what might be causing this pain. Are there any tests you would recommend to help us figure it out?"

4. **Finally, seek their opinion.** Invite your doctor to share their thoughts and expertise. You might say, "What do you think is the most likely cause of my symptoms, and how do we rule out other possibilities?"

If your doctor seems dismissive or defensive, do not panic. Go back to creating safety. Reassure them that you trust their opinion but would like them to clarify their reasoning. For example, "I trust your judgment, but I would like to understand why you think it's X. Have other causes been ruled out? Are there any other tests or specialists you would recommend to help us get to the root cause?"

If you are uncertain about the treatment offered, it is okay to not agree to things right away. You can ask questions. You might say, "I understand it may take time to figure things out, but is this treatment necessary right now? Are there less invasive options or natural treatments we could try first?"

You can take a pause. You might ask for more time to think about the options and get back to them with your decision once you have had time to process the information or get a second opinion.

Always schedule a follow-up visit. The first path may need revision, and another plan may need to be created. Your health is a journey, not a one-time event.

You have learned to ask the right questions and communicate your needs clearly. But what comes next? It is time to take action and follow through.

Here are six questions you can ask your doctor to ensure you are getting the care you need:

1. What tests do you recommend based on my symptoms, and what information will they provide?
2. What are the possible diagnoses, and how do we narrow them down?
3. What treatment options are available, and what are the benefits and risks of each?
4. Are there any lifestyle changes or self-care strategies I can try to help manage my symptoms?
5. Should I consult a specialist, and if so, who would you recommend?
6. When should we schedule a follow-up appointment to reassess my progress or adjust the treatment plan?

Amy's story is proof that change is possible. She didn't give up, and neither should you. When you take these steps: knowing yourself, researching your symptoms, and asking for what you need, you are not just advocating for your health. You are reclaiming your power.

So, let me ask you: Are you ready to take charge of your health? Are you ready to speak up, to ask questions, and to demand answers? Because when you do, you are not just helping yourself, you are paving the way for every woman who has ever felt invisible in a doctor's office. And trust me, that is a revolution worth starting.

Final Thoughts

Your voice matters. Remember, your relationship with your doctor is a partnership. It is not about challenging their authority but about working together to find the best path forward. If you ever feel dismissed or unheard, take a deep breath and return to the conscious communication model. Reaffirm your trust in their expertise, restate your concerns, and ask for clarification.

This approach keeps the conversation open and respectful, ensuring that your voice is heard without creating tension. And if you ever feel like your concerns are not being addressed, do not hesitate to seek a second opinion. Your health is too important to settle for anything less than the care you deserve.

By staying informed, organized, and proactive, you are not just advocating for yourself, you are setting an example for others. Your journey can inspire and empower other women to take control of their health, creating a ripple effect of change.

Doctor Visit Preparation Worksheet

Organize Your Thoughts and Make the Most of Your Appointment

Top 3 Things I Want to Discuss Today

1. Primary Concern:
2. Secondary Concern:
3. Tertiary Concern:

Breakdown of Each Concern

Use the following sections to organize your thoughts for each of your top 3 concerns.

History of Present Illness (HPI):

1. When did this issue start?
2. How often does it occur?
3. What does it feel like? (Describe the pain, discomfort, or symptoms in detail.)
4. What makes it better?
5. What makes it worse?
6. Have you noticed any patterns or triggers?

Relevant Past Medical History:

1. Have you had this issue before? If so, when and how was it treated?
2. Do you have any related medical conditions?

Family History:

1. Does anyone in your family have a similar condition or symptoms?

Social History:

1. Are there any lifestyle factors (diet, exercise, stress, sleep, etc.) that might be contributing?

Previous Tests or Diagnoses:

1. Have you had any tests or imaging related to this issue?
2. What were the results?

Medications Tried:

1. What medications, supplements, or treatments have you tried for this issue?
2. Did they help, make it worse, or have no effect?

Additional Questions to Ask My Doctor

Follow-Up Plan

1. What tests or next steps do I need?
2. When should I schedule a follow-up appointment?
3. Are there any lifestyle changes I should make?

Tip: Bring this worksheet to your appointment and share it with your doctor. Being organized will help you make the most of your time and ensure your concerns are addressed.

 *For a complete companion resource, including all "Questions to Discuss with Your Doctor," Supplement Lists, and Guides, scan the QR code.*

Chapter 10

Own Your Health: Advocate, Share, and Empower Each Other

"Communities and countries and ultimately the world are only as strong as the health of their women."

—**Michelle Obama**

Why do so many of us treat our health as optional until it becomes an emergency? What would your life look like if you prioritized your health as much as you prioritize everyone else's?

I want to share a story with you, one that might feel familiar. It is about Lisa, a woman who embodied strength and selflessness. Lisa was a devoted mother of two daughters, one of whom was born with a disability and required constant care. She was the rock of her family, the one who held everything together. Her husband, her parents, her friends, her neighbors, they all leaned on her. She showed up for everyone, every single day, without fail. But in her unwavering dedication to others, she forgot one crucial person: herself.

Then, one day, her younger daughter was diagnosed with cancer. Lisa's world shattered. Yet, even in the face of this devastating news, she felt she had no permission to grieve. Her family needed her to be strong, to take charge, to navigate endless doctor's appointments, research treatments, and travel across the country for the best care. Lisa buried her pain, her fear, and her exhaustion deep inside. She projected strength on the outside, but inside, she was crumbling.

The toll on her health began to show. Her mental health deteriorated, and she turned to alcohol to cope. She was drowning in silence, carrying the weight of the world on her shoulders.

This is where our paths crossed. When I first met Lisa, she told me her family was her entire world, her purpose, her reason for being. I asked her to imagine what would happen if she became seriously ill, or worse, if she was no longer there for them. How would her family survive without her? That question struck a chord. For the first time, Lisa realized that by neglecting her own health, she was not just hurting herself, she was putting her family at risk.

Lisa began to see that she didn't have to do it all alone. She deserved rest, healing, and care just as much as anyone else. Taking care of herself was not selfish, it was the most selfless thing she could do for her family.

This realization became the catalyst for change in Lisa's life and it can be the starting point for you, too. What would your life look like if you made your health a priority, just as Lisa learned to prioritize her own well-being?

She started by opening up to her family about her struggles, something she had never done before. She carved out time for self-care, no longer viewing it as a luxury but as a necessity. She began a meditation practice to quiet her mind and hired a Pilates instructor to rebuild her physical strength. She reconnected with her friends, her tribe, and allowed herself to lean on their collective support and love.

Lisa gave herself permission to slow down. She focused on her health, making better food choices, prioritizing sleep, and using mindfulness to navigate stressful situations. As she began to heal, she noticed a profound shift. She was more present for her daughters, her husband, and her family. She had more energy, more patience, and more joy to give.

This shift in perspective didn't just improve her life, it transformed her approach to everything. The changes she made to care for herself radiated outward, touching every part of her family and every aspect of her life. How might taking small steps for yourself lead to similar transformation in your life?

But Lisa's journey did not stop there. Her experience caring for her eldest daughter inspired her to help other families facing similar challenges. She recognized a gap in resources for adults with disabilities and turned her pain into purpose by founding a nonprofit organization to support them. She also created a support group for parents of children with disabilities, offering them the understanding and community she had once longed for.

Lisa's story is a powerful reminder that self-care is not selfish, it is essential. By prioritizing her own health and well-being, she not only transformed her life but also created a legacy of love, support, and empowerment for her family and her community. She gave her family the greatest gift of all: a healthy, present, and thriving mother.

Lisa's journey shows us that even amid life's greatest challenges, we have the power to choose ourselves. And in doing so, we become better for everyone we love.

Why Survive When You Can Thrive Through Health?

Let us do a quick activity together. Imagine your life five years from now. You have decided today that your health is a priority. You have taken small steps to care for yourself, whether it is scheduling that overdue doctor's appointment, setting boundaries at work, making better food choices, joining a gym, or simply permitting yourself to rest. You see yourself traveling, enjoying time with your loved ones, staying independent, and feeling physically and mentally fit. Most of all, you feel joyful and content.

What does that future look like for you? How does it feel?

Hold onto that vision. That is the future you have the power to create. That is the future where you are not just surviving, you are thriving.

So, now that you have envisioned a healthier you, what is one small step you can take today to prioritize your health? Maybe it is scheduling that mammogram you have been putting off. Maybe it is setting aside 10 minutes a day to meditate or go for a walk. Maybe it is simply giving yourself permission to say no to something that drains you.

Whatever it is, write it down. Take out your phone or even a scrap of paper and write it down. This is your commitment to yourself. This is your first step toward a future where your health is not an afterthought, it is a priority.

And remember, you do not have to do this alone. Women are tribal by nature. We thrive in communities. Share your commitment with someone you trust. Let them hold you accountable. Let them cheer you on.

When you prioritize your health, you are not just changing your own life, you are setting an example for every woman around you. You are showing them that it is okay to put themselves first. You are showing them that their health matters.

Making the One-on-One Connection

Women have an incredible ability to uplift and validate each other. Think about the last time a friend confided in you about her health struggles. Did you listen? Did you offer support? That is advocacy in action. It is in these moments of connection that we realize how powerful our shared experiences can be. When we open up to one another, we create a space where vulnerability is met with understanding, and pain is met with compassion. These connections are lifelines, reminders that we are not alone in our struggles.

While we are often quick to offer support to others, many of us struggle to receive it in return. We tell ourselves we do not want to burden anyone, or that we should be able to handle everything on our own. I have been there, too. When I was going through my cancer appointments, surgeries and treatments, I felt I needed to do it alone. I have sat in doctor's offices as the patient, carrying my own fears silently, thinking I had to be the strong one. But let me tell you something I have learned through my own journey and through the stories of countless women I have worked with, allowing yourself to receive support is not a sign of weakness, it is an act of strength. It is saying, "I matter, too."

And when you permit yourself to receive, you create a beautiful cycle of giving and receiving.

Another way of making a meaningful connection is through mentoring. If you have navigated the healthcare system, learned to advocate for yourself, or found solutions to your health challenges, you have wisdom to share. Younger women, or those just starting their health journeys, need guidance. They need to hear your story, the struggles, the triumphs, and the lessons learned along the way. By mentoring others, you can help them avoid the pitfalls you faced and empower them to take control of their health.

I have seen the transformative power of mentorship in my own practice. I have had the pleasure of helping women in medicine, who are feeling overwhelmed, balancing long work hours with a family, feeling lost and overwhelmed, and looking for hope and direction through the guidance of someone who has walked a similar path. And as the mentor, I have found healing and purpose in the act of giving back. It is a reminder that our struggles are not in vain, they can become a source of strength for others.

So, I encourage you to seek out those authentic connections in your life. Find the people who lift you up, who listen without judgment, and who remind you of your worth. And when you are ready, extend that same kindness to someone else. Whether it is through a formal mentorship or simply being there for a friend, your voice and your story have the power to change lives.

Together, we can create a world where no woman has to navigate her health journey alone. Where every woman feels seen, heard, and supported. And where our collective strength becomes a force for healing and empowerment.

You are not alone. And you are so deeply needed. Let us lift each other up, one connection at a time.

Making the One-to-Many Connection

Now, imagine that same kindness and solidarity on a larger scale. Picture a network of women, sharing their stories, and offering support in ways that ripple out far beyond their own lives. This is the power of community, a force that can transform not just individual lives, but entire systems of care and understanding.

Finding and connecting with support groups, whether online or offline, can be life changing. These communities are safe spaces where you can share your story, ask questions, and find comfort in knowing others understand what you are going through. I have made it part of my mission to hold space in my office classroom for educational sessions, virtual meetings, and mind-body practice sessions. A place where women who felt isolated and overwhelmed find a sense of belonging and hope in these groups. Whether it is a Facebook group for women managing chronic pain, a local meetup for new moms navigating postpartum health, or a virtual support circle for those dealing with infertility or cancer, these spaces remind us that we are not alone.

Social platforms or local meetups can connect you with women who have faced similar challenges. These groups are more than just a place to vent, they are a source of empowerment, resources, and hope. They are where you can learn about treatments that worked for others, get the names of trusted doctors, discover new ways to advocate for yourself, and even find the courage to try something you have been hesitant about. They are where you can celebrate small victories and find solace during setbacks.

And do not underestimate the power of sharing your own story. When you open up about your experiences, you give others permission to do the same. You become a beacon of strength for someone else who might be struggling in silence. I have seen patients heal in ways they never expected after they shared their journey, whether it was about overcoming a health crisis, navigating menopause, or managing mental health. It is as if by speaking their truth, they reclaimed a piece of themselves they thought they had lost.

But let us take this even further. Imagine what happens when these stories and connections grow into something bigger. When women come together to advocate for better research, more funding, and systemic changes in healthcare. When we use our collective voices to demand that our pain, our symptoms, and our experiences are taken seriously. This is where real change happens.

I have seen women in support groups go on to start nonprofits, lead advocacy campaigns, and even influence policy changes. They have turned their pain into purpose, and in doing so, they have created a legacy of care and empowerment for generations to come. You have that power, too. Your story, your voice, your presence in these communities, it all matters.

So, I encourage you to seek out these spaces. Whether it is online or in person, find the group that feels right for you. Share your story when you are ready and listen to others with an open heart. And remember, you are not just a participant in these communities, you are a vital part of them. Your courage to show up, to share, and to connect has the power to change lives. Including your own.

Mentorship is powerful, but collective action is transformative. When women unite in support groups, advocacy, or nonprofits, they turn pain into purpose, creating ripples that reshape policies, culture, and healthcare access. This is how local movements spark global change.

Making a Global Impact

Being a woman in this world is both a beautiful and complex experience. Across the globe, we face unique challenges when it comes to accessing healthcare and achieving the health outcomes we deserve. These challenges may look different depending on where we live, our cultural backgrounds, our sexual orientations, or our financial circumstances, but at the heart of it, there is a shared thread that connects us all.

I want you to know that your struggles, your fears, and your hopes are valid. Whether you have faced barriers to care, felt unheard in a doctor's office, or worried about the health of someone you love, you are not alone. So many women carry similar burdens, and yet, there is strength in this shared experience. It is a strength that can unite us, inspire us, and drive us to create change.

Imagine, for a moment, the power you hold within you. By taking action, whether it is advocating for better healthcare policies, supporting organizations that uplift women's health, or simply sharing your story, you can create ripples that extend far beyond your own life. These ripples can reach women in your community, across the country, and even around the world. Women you may never meet could one day benefit from the changes you help bring about. Their lives could be touched by your courage, your voice, and your determination to make a difference.

You might be wondering, 'How can I make a difference? The answer lies in taking small actions that can have a profound impact. You do not have to do it all at once, and you do not have to do it alone. Together, as women supporting women, we can break down barriers, challenge injustices, and build a world where every woman has the opportunity to thrive. Look at some of the ways you can make an impact.

1. Participate in Clinical Trials

Clinical trials are essential for advancing medical knowledge, yet women are often underrepresented in them. By participating, you can help researchers better understand how diseases affect women and develop treatments tailored to our needs. To find trials near you, visit trusted resources like ClinicalTrials.gov or check with local hospitals and universities. Your involvement could lead to breakthroughs that save lives.

2. Donate to Women's Health Research

Financial support is critical for advancing research into conditions that disproportionately affect women. Consider donating to organizations like the Society for Women's Health Research (swhr.org), the Endometriosis Foundation of America (endofound.org), or the Lupus Research Alliance (lupusresearch.org). Even small contributions can make a big difference. Every dollar you give helps fund studies that could change the way we understand and treat women's health conditions.

3. Advocate for Funding and Policy Change

Your voice matters to policymakers. Write to your representatives, sign petitions, and join advocacy campaigns that push for increased funding for women's health research. Organizations like Women's Health Access Matters (WHAM) (thewhamreport.org) provide tools and resources to help you take action. Let your representatives know that women's health is a priority, your advocacy can help ensure they receive the attention and resources it deserves.

4. Share Your Data Responsibly

Some research initiatives collect health data from women to identify patterns and trends. For example, the Apple Women's Health Study (apple.com/apple-womens-health-study) allows women to contribute data from their Apple Watches to help researchers better understand menstrual cycles, fertility, and more. Look for similar opportunities to share your health data responsibly through trusted institutions. Your information could help uncover insights that lead to better care for all women.

5. Educate Yourself and Others

The more you know about the gaps in women's health research, the better equipped you will be to advocate for change. Seek out evidence-based resources like the Office on Women's Health (womenshealth.gov) or peer-reviewed journals. Share what you learn with your community and encourage others to get involved. Knowledge is power, and when we educate ourselves and others, we create a collective force for change.

6. Raise Awareness Through Your Platform

Social media and other platforms have given us a megaphone to amplify women's health issues. Use your voice to share research, challenge misconceptions, and advocate for change. Post about your experiences, share articles, or start conversations about conditions that are often misunderstood or ignored. When you speak up, you give others the courage to do the same.

7. Support Local and Global Initiatives

Look for local organizations or global initiatives that focus on women's health. Volunteer your time, donate supplies, or simply spread the word about their work. Groups like Global Alliance for Women's Health (GAWH) and The Pan American Health Organization (PAHO) are pushing for a broader lens, ensuring conditions like heart disease, depression, and autoimmune disorders receive equitable attention in global health agendas.

The Bigger Picture

Imagine a world where every woman, no matter where she lives, has access to the care and support she deserves. A world where conditions like endometriosis, fibromyalgia, and lupus are no longer dismissed or misunderstood. A world where women's health is a priority, not an afterthought.

This is the world we are working toward, and you have a role to play in creating it. Your story, your voice, and your actions matter. Whether it is participating in a clinical trial, donating to research, or simply sharing your experiences, you are contributing to a movement that is changing lives.

So, let us dream bigger. Let us push harder. Let us demand the care, the research, and the respect we deserve. Together, we can create a future where every woman's health is valued, understood, and prioritized.

Final Thoughts

I wrote this book for you, to empower you to take charge of your health. Your health journey begins with you. Trust your instincts, track your symptoms, and do not be afraid to speak up. Refuse to accept dismissive answers or inadequate care. You are your own best advocate. Your body speaks a language only you can fully understand. Listen to it. Honor it. Fight for it. You are not just a patient; you are a partner in your care and a warrior in your story.

But your power does not end with yourself. Share your story, whether with a friend, a support group, or on social media. Your experiences can inspire and educate others. Advocate for systemic changes in healthcare to ensure no woman is left behind. When you speak your truth, you give others permission to do the same. Your voice has the power to shift narratives, challenge outdated systems, and create a future where women's health is no longer an afterthought.

The ripple effect is real. When you take control of your health, you empower your family, your community, and society as a whole. Imagine a future where women's health is prioritized, understood, and respected. A future where diseases like endometriosis, autoimmune disorders, and fibromyalgia are met with the research, funding, and compassion they deserve. A future where no woman has to fight to be heard or beg for answers. That future starts with you.

As we come to the end of this chapter and this book, I want you to know this: You are not alone. Your struggles, your triumphs, and your voice matter. Think about everything we have explored together: how diseases affect women differently, the importance of advocating for yourself, the power of supporting other women, and the impact we can make in our communities and beyond. These are not just ideas;

they are calls to action. They are invitations to step into your power, to use your voice, and to be part of something bigger than yourself.

So, my dear reader, own your health. Share your story. Empower each other. Lift up the women around you and let them lift you up in return. Together, we can create a world where every woman's voice is heard, and every woman's health matters.

This is not just a dream; it is a possibility. And it starts with you.

With love and unwavering belief in you,

—Jyoti Patel, MD

Appendix A

The ACE Test

The ACE (Adverse Childhood Experiences) Score is a tool used to measure the impact of traumatic or stressful experiences during childhood on long-term health and well-being. The score is based on the original Adverse Childhood Experiences Study conducted by the CDC and Kaiser Permanente.[66] Each "yes" answer to the questions below adds 1 point to your ACE score, with a maximum score of 10.

ACE Score Questionnaire

1. Before your 18th birthday, did a parent or other adult in the household often or very often swear at you, insult you, put you down, or humiliate you?
    - ☐ Yes = 1 point
    - ☐ No = 0 points
    - ☐ Physical Abuse:

2. Before your 18th birthday, did a parent or other adult in the household often or very often push, grab, slap, or throw something at you? Or ever hit you so hard that you had marks or were injured?

   ☐ Yes = 1 point
   ☐ No = 0 points
   ☐ Sexual Abuse:

3. Before your 18th birthday, did an adult or person at least five years older than you ever touch or fondle you or have you touch their body in a sexual way? Or attempt or actually have oral, anal, or vaginal intercourse with you?

   ☐ Yes = 1 point
   ☐ No = 0 points
   ☐ Emotional Neglect:

4. Before your 18th birthday, did you often or very often feel that no one in your family loved you or thought you were important or special? Or that your family didn't look out for each other, feel close to each other, or support each other?

   ☐ Yes = 1 point
   ☐ No = 0 points
   ☐ Physical Neglect:

5. Before your 18th birthday, did you often or very often feel that you didn't have enough to eat, had to wear dirty clothes, and had no one to protect you? Or that your parents were too drunk or high to take care of you or take you to the doctor if you needed it?

   ☐ Yes = 1 point
   ☐ No = 0 points
   ☐ Parental Separation or Divorce:

6. Before your 18th birthday, was a biological parent ever lost to you through divorce, abandonment, or other reason?
    - ☐ Yes = 1 point
    - ☐ No = 0 points

7. Before your 18th birthday, was your mother or stepmother often or very often pushed, grabbed, slapped, or had something thrown at her? Or sometimes, often, or very often kicked, bitten, hit with a fist, or hit with something hard? Or ever repeatedly hit over at least a few minutes or threatened with a gun or knife?
    - ☐ Yes = 1 point
    - ☐ No = 0 points
    - ☐ Household Substance Abuse:

8. Before your 18th birthday, did you live with anyone who was a problem drinker or alcoholic, or who used street drugs?
    - ☐ Yes = 1 point
    - ☐ No = 0 points
    - ☐ Household Mental Illness:

9. Before your 18th birthday, was a household member depressed or mentally ill, or did a household member attempt suicide?
    - ☐ Yes = 1 point
    - ☐ No = 0 points
    - ☐ Incarcerated Household Member:

10. Before your 18th birthday, did a household member go to prison?
    - ☐ Yes = 1 point
    - ☐ No = 0 points

Calculating Your ACE Score

Add up the number of "yes" answers. Your total score will range from 0 to 10.

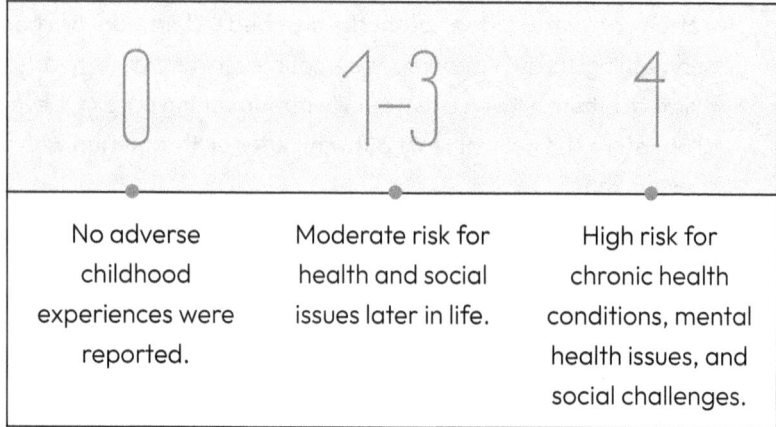

0	1-3	4
No adverse childhood experiences were reported.	Moderate risk for health and social issues later in life.	High risk for chronic health conditions, mental health issues, and social challenges.

What Does Your ACE Score Mean?

The ACE score is not a diagnosis or a definitive predictor of future outcomes, but it highlights the potential impact of childhood trauma on physical and mental health. Higher ACE scores are associated with increased risks for:

- Chronic health conditions (e.g., heart disease, diabetes)
- Mental health issues (e.g., depression, anxiety)
- Substance abuse
- Relationship difficulties
- Lower life expectancy

If you have a high ACE score, it is important to seek support from mental health professionals, counselors, or support groups to address the long-term effects of childhood trauma. Healing and resilience are possible with the right resources and care.

For a complete companion resource, including all "Questions to Discuss with Your Doctor," Supplement Lists, and Guides, scan the QR code.

Appendix B

Recommended Supplements for Lasting Health

Supplements can be a helpful addition to your wellness toolkit, especially when paired with a healthy lifestyle and personalized care. Whether you are supporting heart health, improving brain function, managing mental health, enhancing your immune system, or strengthening bones, muscles, and joints, these evidence-based supplements can provide extra support. By focusing on specific health areas such as cardiovascular, cognitive, emotional well-being, immune function, and musculoskeletal health, you can make a significant difference in your overall health in small, targeted steps. These supplements are meant to complement a broader strategy that includes proper nutrition, lifestyle changes, and personalized care. As always, consult your healthcare provider before starting any new supplement, especially if you are managing an autoimmune condition or taking medications.

Chapter 2: Suggested Supplements for Hormone Health

Hormone health is essential for overall well-being, influencing everything from energy levels and mood to metabolism and reproductive health. While lifestyle factors like diet, exercise, and stress management play a key role, certain evidence-based supplements can help support hormonal balance. Always consult your healthcare provider before starting any new supplement, especially if you have a medical condition or are taking medications.

Here are some of the most well-researched supplements for hormone health:

1. **Vitamin D:** 1,000 - 5,000 IU/day based on labs. May help insulin sensitivity, inflammation and improve ovulation.
2. **Magnesium Glycinate:** 200mg -400mg/day. May help with insulin resistance, stress, sleep, and PMS.
3. **Omega-3 Fatty Acids:** 1-3gm/day may help reduce inflammation, support hormone balance and improve lipid profile.
4. **Myo-Inositol:** 2-4g/day may improve insulin sensitivity, PCOS and cycles.
5. **Adaptogens:** (Ashwagandha 300- 600 mg/d may help reduce cortisol and support thyroid function, Rhodiola 200-400mg/d may boost energy and reduce fatigue, Shatavari 500–1,000 mg/day) may help with libido, energy, mood, and stress.
6. **B Vitamins (B6, B12, Folate):** May help with metabolizing estrogen and energy.
7. **Vitex (Chasteberry):** 400mg -500mg/day. May help with PMS and irregular cycles.
8. **Maca Root:** 1.5gm -3gm/day. May help with libido and energy.

9. **Evening Primrose Oil:** 1gm - 1.5mg/day. May help with hot flashes.
10. **DIM (Diindolylmethane):** 100mg -200mg/day. Helps with estrogen dominance.
11. **Probiotics:** Helps with hormone regulation and detoxification.

Chapter 3: Ten Suggested Supplements for Heart Health

For heart disease, certain evidence-based supplements have shown clear benefits in supporting heart health. However, it's important to note that supplements should never replace prescribed medications or lifestyle changes.

1. **Omega-3 Fatty Acids (Fish Oil):** 1-4gm/day.

    EP and DHA can reduce triglycerides and lower inflammation.

2. **Coenzyme Q10 (CoQ10):** 100mg-300mg/day.

    May improve symptoms of heart failure, improve blood pressure, and heart function.

3. **Magnesium Taurate:** 200mg- 400mg/day.

    May improve blood pressure, regulate heart rhythm, and relax blood vessels.

4. **Garlic Extract:** 600mg- 1200mg/day.

    May slow the progression of plaque buildup in the arteries, lower blood pressure, and improve LDL cholesterol.

5. **Plant Sterols and Stanols:** 2gm/day.

    May help lower LDL cholesterol.

6. **Fiber Supplements (Psyllium):** 5-10gm/day.

    May help lower LDL cholesterol and improve blood sugar.

7. **L-Carnitine**: 1-3gm/day.

   May help improve symptoms of heart failure and improve exercise tolerance.

8. **Vitamin D**: 1,000-5,000 IU/day depending on blood levels.

   May reduce the risk of heart attacks and stroke.

9. **Hawthorn Extract**: 160mg -900mg/day (2-3% std. flavonoid)

   May improve blood flow, lower blood pressure, and reduce symptoms of heart failure.

10. **Green Tea Extract (EGCG):** 250mg -500mg/day.

    May improve LDL cholesterol and endothelial function.

Always consult with a healthcare provider before starting any new supplement regimen, especially if you have underlying health conditions, are taking medications, or are pregnant/nursing.

Chapter 4: Suggested Supplements for Brain Health

Supporting your brain health goes beyond diet and exercise. Certain evidence-based supplements have shown promise in supporting cognitive function, protecting against age-related decline, and reduce the risk of neurodegenerative diseases like Alzheimer's. However, these supplements should not replace a healthy lifestyle, but they can serve as powerful allies in your wellness toolkit. As always, consult your healthcare provider before starting any new supplement, especially if you have any underlying conditions or take medications.

Here are some of the most promising supplements for cognitive support:

1. **Omega-3 Fatty Acids** (DHA and EPA): 1-2 grams daily of DHA and EPA

May help with cognitive performance and help slow age-related decline.

2. **Phosphatidylserine** (PS): 100-300mg daily

    May improve memory, focus, and cognition.

3. **Acetyl-L-Carnitine** (ALCAR): 500mg-2gm daily

    May improve memory, mood, and focus.

4. **Vitamin B Complex** (B6, B9/folate, and B12):
    - B6 (Pyridoxine): 10-50mg daily (higher doses should be monitored).
    - B9 (Methyl Folate): 400-800mcg daily
    - B12 (Methyl cobalamin): 500-2000mcg daily

May improve memory, reduce brain atrophy, and support neurotransmitter function.

1. **Vitamin D**: 1,000-5,000 IU daily

    May protect against cognitive decline.

2. **Curcumin** (Turmeric Extract) with black pepper: 500mg-1000mg per day

    May improve cognitive function and reduce amyloid plaques in the brain.

3. **Bacopa Monnieri**: 300mg-600mg daily

    May improve memory and cognition.

4. **Lion's Mane Mushroom**: 500mg-1gm daily

    May help mild cognitive impairment.

5. **Magnesium L-Threonate**: 1.5gm-2gm daily

    Crosses the blood-brain barrier and may help with brain aging and cognitive function.

6. **Alpha-GPC**: 300mg- 600mg daily

    May help improve cognition in moderate dementia.

Always consult with a healthcare provider before starting any new supplement regimen, especially if you have underlying health conditions, are taking medications, or are pregnant/nursing.

From Chapter 5: Suggested Supplements for Mental Health

1. **Omega-3 Fatty Acids** (DHA and EPA): 1-2 grams per day

   Supports brain health, reduces inflammation, and may improve mood and reduce symptoms of depression and anxiety.

2. **Magnesium Glycinate**: 200-400 mg daily

   Helps calm the nervous system, reduces stress, and improves sleep quality.

3. **Vitamin D**: 1,000-2,000 IU daily (or higher if deficient)

   Supports mood regulation and may reduce symptoms of depression—especially in those with low levels.

4. **B Vitamins** (B6, B9, and B12):
   - B6 (Pyridoxine): 10-50mg daily (higher doses should be monitored)
   - B9 (Methyl Folate): 400-800mcg daily
   - B12 (Methyl cobalamin): 500-2000mcg daily

   May improve memory, reduce brain atrophy, and support neurotransmitter function.

   Support energy production, neurotransmitter synthesis, and mood regulation.

5. **Probiotics**: 10-20 billion CFUs daily

   Psychobiotics support the gut-brain axis, reduce anxiety, and improve mood.

6. **L-Theanine**: 100–200 mg daily

    Promotes relaxation, reduces anxiety, and improves focus—without causing drowsiness.

7. **Ashwagandha**: 300–500 mg daily

    An adaptogen that helps regulate cortisol levels, reduce stress and improve overall well-being.

8. **Zinc**: 15–30 mg daily

    Supports brain function and mood regulation; deficiencies are linked to depression and anxiety.

9. **Saffron**: 30 mg daily

    May boost mood and reduce symptoms of mild to moderate depression.

10. **NAC (N-Acetyl Cysteine):** 600–1,200 mg daily

    An antioxidant that supports brain health, reduces oxidative stress, and may improve symptoms of depression and OCD.

    Always consult with a healthcare provider before starting any new supplement regimen, especially if you have underlying health conditions, are taking medications, or are pregnant/nursing.

From Chapter 6: Supplements to Support Immune Health Against Infections

Suggested Supplements to Fight Infections

1. **Vitamin D:** 2,000–5,000 IU per day

    Essential for immune function and may reduce susceptibility to infections.

2. **Vitamin C:** 500–1,000 mg per day

    Supports immune cell function and may reduce the severity and duration of infections.

3. **Zinc:** 15–30 mg per day

    Critical for immune cell development and may shorten the duration of colds.

4. **Elderberry:** Follow label instructions (typically 1–2 teaspoons of syrup or 1–2 capsules daily)

    May reduce the severity and duration of viral infections like the flu.

5. **Probiotics:** 10–50 billion CFUs per day

    Supports gut health and immune function by balancing gut bacteria.

6. **Echinacea:** Follow label instructions (typically 300–500 mg daily)

    May boost immunity and reduce the risk of catching a cold.

7. **Selenium:** 100–200mcg per day

    Enhances antioxidant defense and immune response.

8. **Quercetin:** 500-1,000mg per day

   Antiviral, stabilizes mast cells, improves zinc uptake.

9. **Andrographis:** 400-600mg per day

   Speeds recovery from colds and flu.

10. **Beta Glucans:** 250-500mg per day

    Activates macrophages and natural killer cells to fight pathogens.

Suggested Supplements to Support Immune Health in Autoimmunity

1. **Omega-3 Fatty Acids** (EPA and DHA): 1,000-3,000 mg per day.

   Anti-inflammatory and may help reduce autoimmune flare-ups.

2. **Curcumin** (Turmeric Extract): 500-1,000 mg per day with black pepper.

   Potent anti-inflammatory that may reduce autoimmune-related inflammation.

3. **Vitamin D**: 2,000-5,000 IU per day.

   Regulates immune function and may reduce autoimmune activity.

4. **Probiotics**: 10-50 billion CFUs per day.

   Supports gut health and may modulate immune responses in autoimmune conditions.

5. **N-Acetylcysteine** (NAC): 600-1,200 mg per day.

   Supports glutathione production, reducing oxidative stress and inflammation.

6. **Quercetin**: 500-1,000 mg per day.

   Antioxidant and anti-inflammatory that may stabilize mast cells and reduce flare-ups.

7. **Resveratrol**: 100-500 mg per day.

   Antioxidant with anti-inflammatory properties that may modulate immune responses.

   Always consult with a healthcare provider before starting any new supplement regimen, especially if you have underlying health conditions, are taking medications, or are pregnant/nursing.

Chapter 7: Suggested Supplements for Digestive Health

1. **Probiotics**: 10-50 billion CFUs per day.

   Helps balance gut bacteria, supports healthy digestion, and may alleviate symptoms of bloating, constipation, and IBS. Look for strains like Lactobacillus and Bifidobacterium.

2. **Digestive Enzymes**: Take with meals as directed on the label.

   Supports the breakdown of food, especially for those with low stomach acid or difficulty digesting fats, proteins, or carbs. Commonly includes amylase, lipase, and protease.

3. **Fiber** (Psyllium Husk or Ground Flaxseed): 5-10 grams per day.

   Promotes regular bowel movements and feeds beneficial gut bacteria. Start with a lower dose and increase gradually to avoid bloating.

4. **Magnesium Citrate or Glycinate**: 200-400 mg per day.

Helps relax the muscles of the digestive tract and can ease constipation. Magnesium glycinate is gentler on the stomach for those with sensitivity.

5. **L-Glutamine**: 5–10 grams per day.

   Supports the repair of the gut lining and may help with conditions like leaky gut or IBS.

6. **Ginger Root Extract**: 250–500 mg per day.

   Reduces nausea, supports healthy digestion, and may ease bloating and cramping.

7. **Peppermint Oil** (Enteric-Coated): 0.2–0.4 mL per day.

   Helps relax the muscles of the digestive tract and may relieve symptoms of IBS, including bloating and abdominal pain.

8. **Slippery Elm Bark**: Follow label instructions (typically 400–500 mg capsules 2–3 times daily).

   Soothes the digestive tract and may help with heartburn, IBS, and inflammation.

9. **Aloe Vera Juice**: 1/4–1/2 cup per day.

   Supports gut healing and may ease symptoms of acid reflux or constipation.

10. **Omega-3 Fatty Acids** (Fish Oil or Algal Oil): 1,000–3,000 mg per day.

    Reduces inflammation in the gut and supports overall digestive health.

11. **Chamomile Extract or Tea**: 1–2 cups of tea or 400–500 mg of extract daily.

    Calms the digestive system, reduces inflammation, and may ease symptoms of IBS or indigestion.

12. **Vitamin D**: 2,000-5,000 IU per day.

    Supports gut health by modulating the immune system and reducing inflammation in the digestive tract.

13. **Zinc Carnosine**: 50-75 mg per day.

    Promotes gut lining repair and may help with conditions like leaky gut or gastritis.

14. **Apple Cider Vinegar** (with the Mother): 1-2 tablespoons diluted in water before meals. May improve digestion by increasing stomach acid production and supporting nutrient absorption.

    Always consult with a healthcare provider before starting any new supplement regimen, especially if you have underlying health conditions, are taking medications, or are pregnant/nursing.

Chapter 8: Suggested Supplements for Bone Health

Suggested Supplements for Bone Health

1. **Calcium**: 1,000-1,200 mg/day.

   Essential for maintaining bone density and strength. Best absorbed when paired with vitamin D.

2. **Vitamin D:** 1,000-5,000 IU/day (based on blood levels).

   Enhances calcium absorption and supports bone mineralization.

3. **Magnesium**: 200-400 mg/day.

   Plays a key role in bone formation and helps regulate calcium levels in the body.

4. **Vitamin K2** (MK-7): 90–180 mcg/day.

   Directs calcium to the bones and teeth, reducing the risk of arterial calcification.

5. **Collagen** (Hydrolyzed): 10–15 gm/day.

   Supports bone matrix structure and may improve bone density over time.

6. **Boron**: 3–5 mg/day.

   Enhances the utilization of calcium, magnesium, and vitamin D for bone health.

7. **Strontium** (Strontium Citrate or Ranelate): 340–680 mg/day.

   May improve bone density and reduce fracture risk (use under medical supervision).

8. **Silica** (Orthosilicic Acid): 10–25 mg/day.

   Supports collagen production and bone mineralization.

9. **Zinc**: 15–30 mg/day.

   Essential for bone tissue repair and regeneration.

10. **Phosphorus**: 700–1,250 mg/day (from food or supplements).

    Works with calcium to build and maintain strong bones.

Suggested Supplements for Muscle Health

1. **Omega-3 Fatty Acids** (Fish Oil): 1–4 gm/day.

   EPA and DHA reduce inflammation, support muscle recovery, and improve muscle protein synthesis.

2. **Creatine Monohydrate:** 3–5 gm/day.

   Enhances muscle strength, power, and lean muscle mass by increasing ATP production.

3. **Branched-Chain Amino Acids** (BCAAs): 5-10 gm/day.

   Supports muscle repair, reduces muscle soreness, and prevents muscle breakdown during exercise.

4. **L-Glutamine**: 5-10 gm/day.

   Aids in muscle recovery, reduces soreness, and supports immune function during intense training.

5. **Magnesium** (Magnesium Glycinate or Citrate): 200-400 mg/day.

   Supports muscle relaxation, reduces cramps, and improves muscle function.

6. **Vitamin D**: 1,000-5,000 IU/day (based on blood levels).

   Enhances muscle strength, reduces inflammation, and supports overall muscle health.

7. **Whey Protein**: 20-40 gm/day.

   Provides essential amino acids to support muscle repair, growth, and recovery post-exercise.

8. **Beta-Hydroxy Beta-Methylbutyrate** (HMB): 2-3 gm/day.

   Reduces muscle breakdown, enhances recovery, and supports lean muscle mass.

9. **Tart Cherry Extract**: 480-1,000 mg/day.

   Reduces muscle soreness and inflammation, improving recovery after intense exercise.

10. **Curcumin** (Turmeric Extract): 500-1,000 mg/day.

    Reduces exercise-induced inflammation and muscle soreness, supporting faster recovery.

Supplements for Joint Health

Joint health is best supported through a combination of proper nutrition, regular low-impact exercise, and targeted supplementation.

1. **Glucosamine Sulfate**: 1,500 mg/day.

    Supports cartilage repair, reduces joint pain, and may slow osteoarthritis progression.

2. **Chondroitin Sulfate**: 800-1,200 mg/day.

    Works synergistically with glucosamine to improve joint flexibility and reduce inflammation.

3. **Omega-3 Fatty Acids** (Fish Oil): 1-4 gm/day.

    EPA and DHA reduce inflammation, easing joint pain and stiffness.

4. **Curcumin** (Turmeric Extract): 500-1,000 mg/day.

    Potent anti-inflammatory properties help reduce joint pain and swelling.

5. **MSM** (Methylsulfonylmethane): 1,500-3,000 mg/day.

    Supports collagen production and reduces joint inflammation.

6. **Collagen** (Hydrolyzed): 10-15 gm/day.

    Promotes cartilage repair and improves joint flexibility and comfort.

7. **Hyaluronic Acid**: 50-200 mg/day.

    Supports joint lubrication and may reduce pain in osteoarthritis.

8. **Boswellia Serrata** (AKBA Extract): 100-250 mg/day.

    Reduces inflammation and improves joint mobility.

9. **Vitamin D**: 1,000-5,000 IU/day (based on blood levels).

    Supports bone and joint health, reducing the risk of joint degeneration.

10. **SAM-e** (S-Adenosylmethionine): 400-1,200 mg/day.

   Supports cartilage repair and reduces joint pain and stiffness.

   Always consult with a healthcare provider before starting any new supplement regimen, especially if you have underlying health conditions, are taking medications, or are pregnant/nursing.

For a complete companion resource, including all "Questions to Discuss with Your Doctor," Supplement Lists, and Guides, scan the QR code.

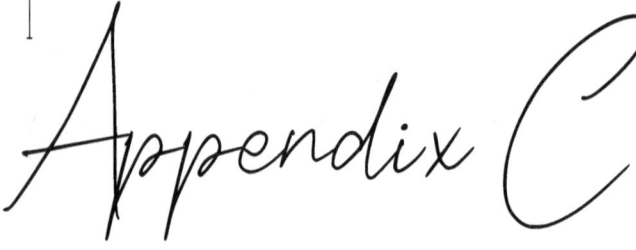

Appendix C

Women's Complete Health Resource Guide

Trusted experts, science-backed tools, and clean-living resources

1. Foundations Of Health

Environmental & Lifestyle Medicine

Experts:
- Dr. Casey Means (@drcaseyskitchen)–Metabolic health
- Dr. Aly Cohen (@thesmarthuman)–Toxin avoidance

Books:
- *Good Energy* by Dr. Casey Means
- *Detoxify* by Dr. Aly Cohen

Tools:
- Non-Toxic Swaps:
  - EWG's Healthy Cleaning Guide

- Home Health:
  - Air: IQAir, Austin Air
  - Water: Berkey Filters
  - Cookware: Caraway, Xtrema
- Product Scanners:
  - Yuka App (yuka.io)-Scans food & cosmetics
  - EWG's Healthy Living App
  - Think Dirty App

2. Hormone Health

Key Physicians:

- Dr. Aviva Romm-Herbal & integrative endocrinology
- Dr. Jolene Brighten-Post-birth control recovery
- Dr. Mary Claire Haver-Menopause nutrition

Must-Reads:

- *Hormone Intelligence* by Dr. Aviva Romm
- *Beyond the Pill* by Dr. Jolene Brighten
- *Estrogen Matters* by Dr. Avrum Bluming

Organizations:

- North American Menopause Society (NAMS)
- PCOS Awareness Association

Research Institutions:

- Monash University Women's Health Research
- NIH Reproductive Sciences Branch

Clinical Trials:

- PCOS Treatment Trials (PCOSChallenge.org)

3. Heart and Metabolic Health

Specialists:

- Dr. Nieca Goldberg–Women's cardiology
- Dr. Suzanne Steinbaum–Preventive cardiology
- Glucose Goddess (@glucosegoddess)–Blood sugar hacks

Research Hubs:

- American Heart Association's Go Red for Women
- Cleveland Clinic Women's Cardiovascular Center

Blood Sugar Tools and Books:

- Levels CGM Program
- Glucose Goddess "10 Hacks" (free download available)
- *Glucose Revolution* by Jessie Inchauspé

Institutions:

- Mayo Clinic Women's Health Center
- Cleveland Clinic Women's Cardiovascular Center

Enrolling in Studies:

- Women's Heart Alliance (AHA-sponsored)
- WISE Study (Cleveland Clinic)
- Women's Heart Study (Brigham & Women's)

4. Brain & Mental Health

Leading Voices:

- Dr. Lisa Mosconi–Alzheimer's prevention
- Dr. Ellen Vora–Anxiety & depression

Resources:

- *The XX Brain* by Lisa Mosconi
- *The Anatomy of Anxiety* by Ellen Vora
- **Apps:**
  - Headspace
  - Calm
  - Nerva (IBS hypnotherapy)

Crisis Support:

- 988 Suicide & Crisis Lifeline
- Postpartum Support International

Research Opportunities

- Women's Alzheimer's Movement Prevention Registry
- Mayo Clinic Women's Cognitive Health Program
- POINTER Study (Alzheimer's prevention)

5. Immune & Autoimmune Health

Pioneers:
- Dr. Terry Wahls-MS & autoimmune protocols
- Dr. Sara Gottfried-Hormone-immune connections

Protocols:
- Wahls Protocol Diet
- The Myers Way (Dr. Amy Myers)

Research:
- Autoimmune Association
- NIH Women's Health Initiative
- Dr. Terry Wahls' MS Clinical Trials
- Autoimmune Association Patient Registry

6. Digestive Health

Top Experts:
- Dr. Amy Myers-Leaky gut & SIBO
- Kayla Barnes, RD-IBS & microbiome

Tools:

- SIBO Info (Dr. Allison Siebecker)
- Nerva App (gut-directed hypnotherapy)
- Monash FODMAP App

GI Research Programs

- Monash University Low FODMAP Diet Studies
- Dr. Siebecker's SIBO Research Registry

7. Muscle, Bone & Joints

Science-Backed Coaches:

- Dr. Stacy Sims–Female athlete physiology
- Dr. Gabrielle Lyon–Muscle-centric medicine

Books:

- *Next Level* by Dr. Stacy Sims
- *Forever Strong* by Dr. Gabrielle Lyon

Bone Health:

- National Osteoporosis Foundation

8. Join Research Studies

1. **Women's Health:** NIH Women's Health Initiative
2. **PCOS:** PCOS Challenge Registry
3. **Alzheimer's:** Women's Alzheimer's Movement

 *For a complete companion resource, including all "Questions to Discuss with Your Doctor," Supplement Lists, and Guides, scan the QR code.*

ABOUT THE AUTHOR

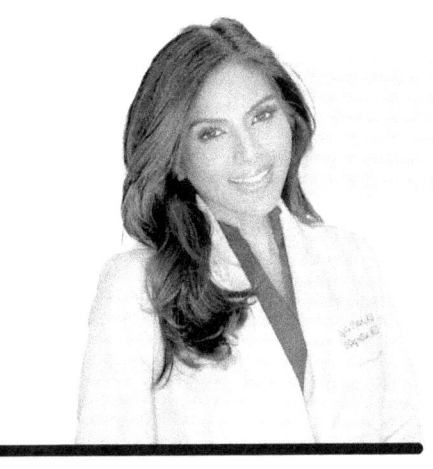

Dr. Jyoti Patel

Dr. Jyoti Patel is a triple board-certified physician in Internal Medicine, Pediatrics, and Integrative Medicine, with additional certification in Functional Medicine. For over twenty years, she has dedicated her career to addressing the unique health challenges women face, combining rigorous medical training with holistic wisdom. Recognized repeatedly as a Top Doctor by *Phoenix Magazine*, Dr. Patel trained under leaders in integrative medicine including Dr. Andrew Weil and Deepak Chopra, developing a sophisticated approach to women's health that looks beyond symptoms to underlying causes.

Specializing in conditions that disproportionately affect women, including hormonal imbalances, autoimmune disorders, and metabolic dysfunction, Dr. Patel brings both scientific precision and deep clinical insight to complex cases often misunderstood in conventional medicine. As a certified teacher of Mindfulness-Based Stress Reduction, she bridges cutting-edge diagnostics with time-tested wellness practices, offering patients comprehensive paths to healing.

Beyond Bikini Medicine reflects Dr. Patel's decades of experience advocating for women's health. The book reveals systemic gaps in medical care while providing actionable strategies for true wellness. Beyond her practice, Dr. Patel has championed community health initiatives including the Fountain Hills Community Garden and mentors the next generation of physicians. She finds balance in desert gardening and family life in Arizona.

Endnotes

1. National Center for Biotechnology Information, *Biology of the Blood-Brain Barrier*, accessed March 20, 2025, https://www.ncbi.nlm.nih.gov/books/NBK236531/.
2. MedStar Health, *Cardiovascular Diagnosis and Research: What You Should Know*, accessed March 20, 2025, https://www.medstarhealth.org/blog/cardiovascular-diagnosis-research.
3. Hopkins Lupus Center, *How Lupus Affects the Cardiovascular System*, accessed March 20, 2025, https://www.hopkinslupus.org/lupus-info/lupus-affects-body/lupus-cardiovascular-system/.
4. Harvard Health Publishing, *Why Are Women More Likely to Develop Alzheimer's Disease?*, accessed March 20, 2025, https://www.health.harvard.edu/blog/why-are-women-more-likely-to-develop-alzheimers-disease-202201202672.
5. Columbia University Journal of Bioethics, *The Bioethical Dimensions of Gender Disparities in Cardiovascular Care*, accessed March 20, 2025, https://journals.library.columbia.edu/index.php/bioethics/article/view/6008.
6. U.S. Government Accountability Office, *Women's Health: Women Face Many Barriers to Health Care*, accessed March 22, 2025, https://www.gao.gov/products/gao-01-286r.
7. U.S. Congress, *S.1 - Health Security Act*, 103rd Congress (1993-1994), accessed March 20, 2025, https://www.congress.gov/bill/103rd-congress/senate-bill/1.
8. Cardiovascular News, *Women 50% More Likely Than Men to Be Given Incorrect Diagnosis Following Heart Attack*, accessed March 20, 2025, https://cardiovascularnews.com/women-50-more-likely-than-men-to-be-given-incorrect-diagnosis-following-heart-attack/.

9. Cathy A. Jenkins et al., "Sex Differences in the Treatment and Outcome of Myocardial Infarction," *The New England Journal of Medicine* 342, no. 16 (2000): 1213–20, accessed March 20, 2025, https://www.nejm.org/doi/full/10.1056/NEJM200004203421603.

10. European Society of Cardiology, *Women More Likely to Die After Heart Attack Than Men*, accessed March 20, 2025, https://www.escardio.org/The-ESC/Press-Office/Press-releases/Women-more-likely-to-die-after-heart-attack-than-men.

11. Healthline, *How Many Cells Are in the Human Body?*, accessed March 20, 2025, https://www.healthline.com/health/number-of-cells-in-body.

12. **Cleveland Clinic**, *Hormones: What They Are, Function & Types*, accessed March 20, 2025, https://my.clevelandclinic.org/health/articles/22464-hormones.

13. **Alzheimer's Association**, *Women and Alzheimer's Disease*, accessed March 20, 2025, https://www.alz.org/alzheimers-dementia/what-is-alzheimers/women-and-alzheimer-s.

14. **Bone Health & Osteoporosis Foundation**, *What Women Need to Know*, accessed March 20, 2025, https://www.bonehealthandosteoporosis.org/preventing-fractures/general-facts/what-women-need-to-know.

15. **Angela H. Ting et al.**, "Sex and Gender in Medical Education: A National Survey of Medical Students' Experiences and Preparedness," *The American Journal of Medicine* 136, no. 9 (September 2023): 1046–54, accessed March 20, 2025, https://www.amjmed.com/article/S0002-9343%2823%2900244-9/fulltext.

16. Centers for Disease Control and Prevention, "About the CDC-Kaiser ACE Study," *Violence Prevention*, last reviewed April 3, 2024, https://www.cdc.gov/violenceprevention/aces/about.html.

17. Cleveland Clinic, "Premenstrual Dysphoric Disorder (PMDD)," *Cleveland Clinic*, last reviewed October 24, 2023, https://my.clevelandclinic.org/health/diseases/9132-premenstrual-dysphoric-disorder-pmdd.
18. Kaitlin Roke et al., "Effect of a Multinutrient Supplement on Mood and Emotional Well-Being in Healthy Adults: A Randomized, Double-Blind, Placebo-Controlled Trial," *Frontiers in Nutrition* 10 (2023): 1228305, https://pmc.ncbi.nlm.nih.gov/articles/PMC10583117/.
19. Rachael Link, "Ashwagandha: What You Need to Know," *Healthline*, July 11, 2023, https://www.healthline.com/nutrition/ashwagandha.
20. National Heart, Lung, and Blood Institute, "Women's Health Initiative (WHI)," *National Heart, Lung, and Blood Institute*, accessed March 20, 2025, https://www.nhlbi.nih.gov/science/womens-health-initiative-whi.
21. "Misinterpretation of WHI Results Decreased Use of Hormones, Even in Women Not at Risk," *Australasian Menopause Society*, last modified January 9, 2019, https://www.menopause.org.au/hp/studies-published/misinterpretation-of-whi-results-decreased-use-of-hormones.
22. Elizabeth Hughes, "Fear of the Dark: Autism, Gender, and the Aesthetics of Engagement," *Autism in Adulthood* 1, no. 1 (2017): 24–33, https://journals.sagepub.com/doi/pdf/10.1177/2053369116680501.
23. Adriana Albini, "20-Year WHI Follow-Up Study Finds Oestrogen Selectively Protects against Breast Cancer in Women Who Have Undergone Hysterectomy," *Cancerworld*, November 2, 2020, https://cancerworld.net/20-year-whi-follow-up-study-finds-oestrogen-selectively-protects-against-breast-cancer-in-women-who-have-undergone-hysterectomy/.
24. Lori A. Bastian, "Hormone Replacement Therapy and the Prevention of Chronic Conditions," *American Family*

Physician 62, no. 8 (October 15, 2000): 1839–46, https://www.aafp.org/pubs/afp/issues/2000/1015/p1839.html.

25. American College of Obstetricians and Gynecologists, "Postmenopausal Estrogen Therapy: Route of Administration and Risk of Venous Thromboembolism," *ACOG Committee Opinion*, no. 556 (April 2013), https://www.acog.org/clinical/clinical-guidance/committee-opinion/articles/2013/04/postmenopausal-estrogen-therapy-route-of-administration-and-risk-of-venous-thromboembolism.

26. JoAnn E. Manson et al., "Menopausal Hormone Therapy and Long-term All-Cause and Cause-Specific Mortality: The Women's Health Initiative Randomized Trials," *JAMA* 318, no. 10 (2017): 927–38, https://jamanetwork.com/journals/jama/fullarticle/2653735.

27. Physicians Committee for Responsible Medicine, *Capital WAVS II: Health Disparities and the Impact of Diet*, 2022, https://pcrm.widen.net/s/kbrn2p6mqx/capital-wavs-ii.

28. Centers for Disease Control and Prevention, "Women and Heart Disease," *Heart Disease*, last reviewed February 5, 2024, https://www.cdc.gov/heart-disease/about/women-and-heart-disease.html.

29. Centers for Disease Control and Prevention, "Women and Heart Disease," *Heart Disease*, last reviewed February 5, 2024, https://www.cdc.gov/heart-disease/about/women-and-heart-disease.html.

30. Avrum Bluming and Carol Tavris, "Hormone Replacement Therapy: Real Concerns and False Alarms," *The Cancer Journal* 26, no. 5 (2020): 417–23, https://pmc.ncbi.nlm.nih.gov/articles/PMC7292717/.

31. Framingham Heart Study, "Framingham Heart Study: Landmark 20th Century Study," *Framingham Heart Study*, accessed March 20, 2025, https://www.framingham.com/heart/4stor_04.htm.

32. American College of Cardiology, "PREDIMED," *American College of Cardiology*, last updated August 8, 2014, https://www.acc.org/Latest-in-Cardiology/Clinical-Trials/2014/08/08/15/35/PREDIMED.
33. American College of Cardiology, "PURE: Just 150 Minutes of Physical Activity Weekly Reduces CV Disease, Deaths," *American College of Cardiology*, September 20, 2017, https://www.acc.org/latest-in-cardiology/articles/2017/09/20/15/26/pure-just-150-minutes-of-physical-activity-weekly-reduces-cv-disease-deaths.
34. Centers for Disease Control and Prevention, "Life Expectancy," *National Center for Health Statistics*, last reviewed February 15, 2024, https://www.cdc.gov/nchs/fastats/life-expectancy.htm.
35. Centers for Disease Control and Prevention, "Alzheimer's Disease," *National Center for Health Statistics*, last reviewed September 13, 2023, https://www.cdc.gov/nchs/fastats/alzheimers.htm.
36. Cleveland Clinic, "What Is Neuroplasticity?" *Cleveland Clinic Health Essentials*, September 13, 2022, https://health.clevelandclinic.org/neuroplasticity.
37.
38. Zia Sherrell, "What to Know About Vagus Nerve Stimulation," Medical News Today, February 27, 2023, https://www.medicalnewstoday.com/articles/326847.
39. Cleveland Clinic, "Serotonin," *Cleveland Clinic*, last reviewed September 11, 2023, https://my.clevelandclinic.org/health/articles/22572-serotonin.

    Deborah M. Mitchell et al., "Prevalence and Predictors of Vitamin D Deficiency in Healthy Adults," *The Journal of Clinical Endocrinology & Metabolism* 82, no. 11 (1997):

3864–71, https://academic.oup.com/jcem/article-abstract/82/11/3864/2866142.

40. Harvard T.H. Chan School of Public Health, "MIND Diet," *The Nutrition Source*, accessed March 20, 2025, https://nutritionsource.hsph.harvard.edu/healthy-weight/diet-reviews/mind-diet/.

41. Helen Lavretsky et al., "A Pilot Study of Yogic Meditation for Family Dementia Caregivers with Depressive Symptoms: Effects on Mental Health, Cognition, and Telomerase Activity," International Journal of Geriatric Psychiatry 28, no. 1 (2013): 57–65, https://pubmed.ncbi.nlm.nih.gov/23332672/.

42. Alzheimer's Research and Prevention Foundation, *The FINGER Study: Summary Report*, 2020, https://alzheimersprevention.org/downloadables/FINGER-study-report-by-ARPF.pdf.

43. Sebastian Köhler et al., "Effect of the MIND Diet Intervention on Cognitive Decline in Older Adults: The MIND Diet Randomized Clinical Trial," Neurology 100, no. 6 (2023): e590–e601, https://www.neurology.org/doi/pdf/10.1212/wnl.0000000000200701.

44. Qian Lin et al., "Tai Chi Chuan and Baduanjin Increase Grey Matter Volume in Older Adults: A Brain Imaging Study," Journal of Alzheimer's Disease 71, no. 2 (2019): 605–14, https://content.iospress.com/articles/journal-of-alzheimers-disease/jad180492.

45. Cyrus A. Raji et al., "Brain Volume in Late Life: Relationship to Fitness and Physical Activity," Journal of Alzheimer's Disease 19, no. 4 (2010): 957–63, https://www.ncbi.nlm.nih.gov/pmc/articles/PMC3000617/.

46. Séverine Sabia et al., "Association of Sleep Duration in Middle and Old Age with Incidence of Dementia," Nature Communications 12 (2021): 2289, https://doi.org/10.1038/s41467-021-22354-2.

47. Lulu Xie et al., "Sleep Drives Metabolite Clearance from the Adult Brain," *Science* 342, no. 6156 (2013): 373–77, https://doi.org/10.1126/science.1241224.
48. Mari Hysing et al., "Screen Time and Sleep Disruption: The Blue Light Effect," *Sleep Medicine Reviews* 47 (2020): 1–10, https://doi.org/10.1016/j.smrv.2019.101216.
49. Alzheimer's Research and Prevention Foundation, "A New Scientific Paper Published About Kirtan Kriya Meditation: Improved Quality of Life," *Alzheimer's Research and Prevention Foundation*, February 23, 2023, https://alzheimersprevention.org/a-new-scientific-paper-published-about-kk-meditation-improved-quality-of-life/.
50. Masashi Nouchi et al., "Lifestyles and Mental Health: A Longitudinal Study of Elderly Japanese People," *Environmental Health and Preventive Medicine* 24, no. 1 (2019): 1–7, https://environhealthprevmed.biomedcentral.com/articles/10.1186/s12199-019-0822-8.
51. Yuda Turana et al., "Lifestyle Intervention for Brain Health: Indonesian MIND Diet Translation, Cultural Adaptation, and Intervention Strategy," *Innovation in Aging* 8, no. 10 (2024): 1–10, https://academic.oup.com/innovateage/article/8/10/igae093/7808678.
52. Joseph A. Hyde et al., "Depression, Anxiety, and Comorbidity in the Canadian Armed Forces," *BMC Psychiatry* 12, no. 1 (2012): 1–11, https://pubmed.ncbi.nlm.nih.gov/22613905/.
53. Bernard Gesch et al., "Influence of Supplementary Vitamins, Minerals and Essential Fatty Acids on the Antisocial Behaviour of Young Adult Prisoners: Randomised, Placebo-Controlled Trial," *The British Journal of Psychiatry* 181, no. 1 (2002): 22–28, https://www.cambridge.org/core/journals/the-british-journal-of-psychiatry/article/influence-of-supplementary-vitamins-minerals-and-essential-fatty-

acids-on-the-antisocial-behaviour-of-young-adult-prisoners/04CAABE56D2DE74F69460D035764A498.

54. University of Illinois at Urbana-Champaign, "Study Links Gut Bacteria to Improved Depression Symptoms," *ScienceDaily*, August 8, 2018, https://www.sciencedaily.com/releases/2018/08/180808193656.htm.

55. National Institutes of Health, "Lack of Sleep Disrupts Brain's Emotional Controls," *NIH Research Matters*, August 27, 2018, https://www.nih.gov/news-events/nih-research-matters/lack-sleep-disrupts-brains-emotional-controls.

56. Liz Mineo, "Over Nearly 80 Years, Harvard Study Has Been Showing How to Live a Healthy and Happy Life," *Harvard Gazette*, April 11, 2017, https://news.harvard.edu/gazette/story/2017/04/over-nearly-80-years-harvard-study-has-been-showing-how-to-live-a-healthy-and-happy-life/.

57. U.S. Department of Health and Human Services, *Our Epidemic of Loneliness and Isolation: The U.S. Surgeon General's Advisory on the Healing Effects of Social Connection and Community*, 2023, https://www.hhs.gov/sites/default/files/surgeon-general-social-connection-advisory.pdf.

58. David A. Merrill et al., "Efficacy of Multimodal, Technology-Supported, and Family-Centered Lifestyle Intervention to Prevent Cognitive Decline in Older Adults: A Randomized Clinical Trial," *JAMA Network Open* 7, no. 2 (2024): e2351261, https://pubmed.ncbi.nlm.nih.gov/38306984/.

59. Ask the Doctors, "Want to Boost Immunity? Look to the Gut," *UCLA Health*, April 19, 2022, https://www.uclahealth.org/news/article/want-to-boost-immunity-look-to-the-gut.

60. Terry Wahls, "About the Wahls Protocol," Terry Wahls, MD, accessed March 22, 2025, https://terrywahls.com/about-the-wahls-protocol/.

61. Carly Cassella, "The Human Digestive System Varies Way More Than We Realize," *ScienceAlert*, July 31, 2022, https://www.sciencealert.com/the-human-digestive-system-varies-way-more-than-we-realize.

    F. Grodstein, G. A. Colditz, and M. J. Stampfer, "Postmenopausal Hormone Use and Cognitive Function in Older Women," *Journal of the American Geriatrics Society* 44, no. 7 (1996): 833–37, https://pubmed.ncbi.nlm.nih.gov/8635705/.

62. Gastro Florida, "IBS Statistics: Gender, Race, and What Else?" *Gastro Florida*, September 21, 2021, https://gastrofl.com/resources/ibs-statistics-gender-race-and-what-else/.

63. UCLA Health, "Want to Boost Immunity? Look to the Gut," *UCLA Health*, April 19, 2022, https://www.uclahealth.org/news/article/want-to-boost-immunity-look-to-the-gut.

64. Amy C. Maher et al., "Sex Differences in Global mRNA Content of Human Skeletal Muscle," *PLoS One* 4, no. 7 (2009): e6335, https://doi.org/10.1371/journal.pone.0006335.

65. Laura Williams, "7 Benefits of High Intensity Interval Training (HIIT)," *Verywell Health*, January 17, 2024, https://www.verywellhealth.com/benefits-of-hiit-8659170.

66. Centers for Disease Control and Prevention, "About the CDC-Kaiser ACE Study," *Violence Prevention*, last reviewed April 3, 2024, https://www.cdc.gov/violenceprevention/aces/about.html.

www.ingramcontent.com/pod-product-compliance
Lightning Source LLC
LaVergne TN
LVHW021807060526
838201LV00058B/3274